BLACK
THERAPISTS
ROCK

A GLIMPSE THROUGH
THE EYES OF EXPERTS

COMPILED BY DERAN YOUNG, LCSW
~ FOREWORD BY LISA SAVAGE PHILLIPS, LCSW ~

Black Therapists Rock: *A Glimpse Through the Eyes of Experts*

Published by Black Therapists Rock, Inc.
blacktherapistsrock.com

ISBN: 978-1-7323565-9-7

Published in the United States of America

This Book is Dedicated to The Village:

PAST: Our ancestors who survived extremely harsh circumstances (leaving intuitive clues), so that we could have a foundation to live life "more abundantly."

PRESENT: Those who have experienced so much pain, that they question their ability to love, and yet are courageous enough to explore the possibilities within their heart and mind.

FUTURE: The youth and unborn children who will be able to live in a world with more compassion, because of the pain we are willing to overcome.

THE MISSION OF BLACK THERAPISTS ROCK

Increasing Awareness of Social & Psychological Issues Impacting Vulnerable Communities and Reducing Stigma Related to Mental Health.

TABLE OF CONTENTS

Showing up...

I had finished graduate school and wore my MSW credentials with a tremendous amount of pride. Having worked hard for that degree, I had the battle scars as proof. I even secured the first job I applied to.

Although I was only 23 years old, I had found someone who believed in me when I struggled to believe in myself.

I was smart and accomplished; yet, the internal negative voices were still loud and believable. The first few years were spent as a newly minted professional in fear. I feared that I lacked life experiences and certainly was inadequate in this mostly "white" space. I clinched to the belief that someday, I would eventually move beyond these insecurities, but I had no idea *how*.

As expected, I was assigned to most of the Black clients, which is not an uncommon occurrence for those of us in the helping professions. I was cool with that, due to there being a level of comfort working with people who looked like me. My clients loved me because of my easily relatable style, and they found support in talking to someone who "understood" them.

Seeing them was my happy place; I could be authentic and not feel judged. The grandmotherly types would bring me cake, call me *sweetheart,* and tell me how much I reminded them of their grand-children.

Was I using social work theory in helping them? Well, probably a mix of theory, intuition, *and* making it up as I went along. Let's be real... it can be difficult to marry theory with practice when you're a new therapist.

So, here's the conflict. When in meetings and social settings with professional colleagues, I wanted to be "unseen." I often sat quietly in the back of the room, hoping to be ignored and wishing for the time to past swiftly so that no one would ask me a question or my opinion. Even as I write this, the painful realization returns.

A bright, young, Black woman, with so much to offer, yet intentionally dimming her bulb and shrinking. The internal struggle was real. Here I was, reveling in the joy and connections I made with my clients, yet sheltering myself from professional relationships, which had the potential of hindering my professional and clinical development.

I felt as if I didn't deserve the adulation of my clients, and ultimately, I had to question my effectiveness with them. I could not continue to split off parts of myself and fully show up for my clients who needed all of me in the therapy room. The path to being a good therapist is the ability to engage in introspection to increase self-awareness. It's the insight gained from internal reflection that improves our ability to help our clients.

When we delve deeper into our psyches and decide to live consciously, we know change has to happen. Otherwise, the internal conflicts will cause mental distress and render us ineffective with our clients and in our own lives.

What was my fix?

Trust me, it didn't come quickly or easily. However, what I needed to do was challenge myself to "show up." To show up for myself and my clients.

What does that mean?

For me, it indicated a need to step outside of self-imposed limitations. I had to deal with the internal, negative voices and confront them head-on. I had to deal with the internalized racism and self-doubt that held my mind captive.

I made the internal shift first by being mindful of my thoughts and core beliefs. I challenged them and ultimately learned how to replace them with more realistic thoughts. Then, I engaged in behavioral shifts. I started sitting *front and center* in meetings. I asked questions and challenged things that didn't make sense to me. I sought out clinical training to improve my effectiveness with my clients and to help bolster my expertise. I also started calling out racism and other 'isms.'

Also, I became an advocate for my clients and used my position to help shape policy for them. I owned my vulnerability, and rather than seeing it as a weakness, I reframed it as my strength.

Here's what I learned: hiding parts of myself reinforced the notion that I didn't belong and that I was an imposter. I also discovered that my internal struggles often mimicked those of my clients. How could I move them through a process that I had not endured? I also learned that I was cheating others, by not allowing them to learn from me. I had a body of knowledge, and albeit limited, experiences that could have benefited others.

Learning how to "show up" helped me to discover a profoundly creative spirit in myself, and I have now nurtured this creativity in developing programs, models, and concepts that have not only proven to be helpful for clients but other professionals as well.

The stories of Black therapists shared in this book are of those who are doing the work to assure that the best of them shows up in the therapy room. They will inspire you to meet *and not shrink* from the challenges unique to Black professionals in this society.

You will learn how they reject boundaries of institutional racism and sexism to rightfully claim their part in professional spaces. You'll find yourself shaking your head in agreement, and at times, shrinking because the story touches an internal place you'd rather not visit. Most importantly, these therapists are showing up and representing what our communities need.

My challenge to other Black mental health professionals is to do the self-work and look for areas where you are holding back parts of yourself. What internal, negative, or self-limiting thoughts are holding you hostage? What do you need to do to *show up* more in your life... and in the lives of your clients?

Our communities need representation and your expertise. We owe it to ourselves, and those in need, to *show up*.

Lisa R. Savage, LCSW
Founder of *The Center for Child Development, Inc*
And the *Delaware Center for Counseling and Wellness, Inc.*

ACKNOWLEDGMENTS

Thousands of people have shown a significant amount of support to us as authors and to Black Therapists Rock as an organization. There is not enough time nor space to express our sincerest gratitude to everyone who played a role in the success of this project. The names below are only a few highlights of individuals and organizations who provided guidance into this work:

To the Authors who bravely stepped up to this challenge; to bare all, in hopes of helping others heal. I'm so proud to stand next to each of you as we do this tremendous work that we have been called to do in our community and ourselves.

Jackee Holder - our first writing coach, who aligned her schedule with ours, all the way from the United Kingdom, to ensure we offered words from an inspired and vulnerable place.

Audra R. Upchurch - my first writing mentor, who taught me how to be fierce with my words, yet gentle in my approach.

Dr. Romeatrius Moss - who was instrumental in the development of Black Therapists Rock as a non-profit organization.

Aprille Franks - who taught me how to leverage our success and our message to reach thousands of people worldwide.

To the community members of **Black Therapists Rock** who continue to help reduce stigma and spread mental health awareness.

To the Center for Self-Leadership for the ongoing support, encouragement, and reminders that "all parts are welcome."

To our clients, families, couples, and individuals, who trust us with their most tender aspects of life and help us grow and learn as a result.

To the children, significant others, mentors, peers, and elders who sustained us along the journey.

Thank you.

INTRODUCTION
By Deran Young, LCSW

When You Think of Trauma, Do You Think of Someone Like Me?

"Owning our story is hard, but not nearly as difficult
as spending our lives running from it."
-Dr. Brené Brown

"Capt. Young, you have Post Traumatic Stress Disorder."
From What? I thought. *My entire life?*

How can that be? I've adapted, I've overcome...
Don't you see how successful I am! I can't have PTSD.

- I do this for a living! I'm a licensed therapist!
- I'm a very engaged & loving mother!
- I'm active in my church and my community!
- I am THE source of strength for my family!
- I'm the one who "made it out"

So what do you MEAN I have PTSD?

My attempts to forget my traumatic childhood and chaotic family dynamics had landed me in this office with a military psychologist telling me things that I just could not agree with.

I'm smart... I had to be smart to take care of my two younger sisters when I myself was just four years old. I was smart enough not to open the door for anyone, just like mama sad. I was smart enough to walk myself to kindergarten, through the maze of housing projects filled with drugs and crime. I was smart enough to get us to the church during the summers where we were able to get a free lunch since school was out. I was smart enough to graduate high school at the age of 17, despite being homeless. I was smart enough to get two masters degrees before the age of 28, while serving full time in the military. I was always told that I was "wise for my age". I've always been able to use my intellect to hide my trauma from others. I was so smart that I finally decided to give in and "play along", just to prove this doctor wrong.

There is no way I could be "sick."

"At present, Capt. Young reports she continues to experience depressed mood nearly every day, poor concentration, low energy, and difficulty falling or staying asleep. Additionally, she endorsed symptoms of anxiety related to an extensive history of trauma related to a sexual assault as well as childhood trauma. Her symptoms include intrusive thoughts, avoidance of thoughts related to the trauma, sleep disturbance, irritability, decreased interest in hobbies or recreational activities, social withdrawal, and difficulty experiencing positive emotions."

As I read through my medical records, it was almost as if they were talking about a completely different person. Someone that I didn't know.

Okay, maybe it's my Thyroid Disorder; once I figure out how to better manage that, I'll be able to return to my home in Italy. I'll be able to pretend like none of this ever happened. That's all I need to do... get up and keep going. Never stop working hard and never look like what you've been through. Just keep trying to be NORMAL...

Yet, every time I thought about returning to my "normal" way of life, I felt exhausted. The truth is, I had been exhausted for a while. What triggered this? Was it the Thyroid Disorder? Or could this be caused by the divorce? Was it the experience in which I had to fight to maintain my highly praised work ethic after reporting to the chain of command that my supervisor called me a N*gga?

Maybe I needed to go back even further...

Was it that, before getting married at 30 years old, I had never heard a man say, "I love you"?

Or even further...

Was it the fact that I desperately joined the military only weeks after graduating high school because I was homeless and hopeless? Was it due to the fact that a military instructor coerced himself into my hotel room just two years prior, and forced me to have sex with him, like it was somehow part of the training curriculum?

No, I think it was much earlier than that...

Was it all the memories of being left on my grandmother's porch in the middle of the night and being told, "I really wish your mother would get off drugs, cuz I'm not raising three more kids. I already raised mine."

Was it watching my sister get a third-degree burn from being forced to put her hand on the stove by our babysitter?

Was it being sexually tortured (i.e., having a broom and other objects shoved up my vagina) for years right under the same roof as my mother, and her never noticing?

Was it being exposed to my mother having sex with various men (audible and one time visually on the living room floor while my sisters and I slept on the couch)?

What the hell do you mean POST traumatic stress?

Living my life was an ongoing effort to block out the trauma, to stay sane, and to focus on surviving day to day. In my mind, there was nothing POST about it; I *had* to keep fighting!

I now realize that even as a mental health professional, I had perpetuated the stigma of mental illness. Who I was professionally, and who I was as a human being, had become so tightly tangled. My accomplishments had become one of the ways that I was running from my story... and myself! I didn't have a true identity; I was only hiding behind the mask of a "competent, well-trained clinician."

Until that point, I don't know if I had many original thoughts of my own because everything had been so heavily influenced by my work, my faith, my role in the community and most of all my FEARS! When I think of generational trauma and legacy burdens, I think of the fear-based beliefs and protective measures that have been passed down.

I feared being alone because it reminded me how lonely I had been during my childhood. So, I made sure that I was always surrounded by people, whether they genuinely cared about me or not.

I feared returning to the days of being hungry and eating food from the trash can, so I ate even when I wasn't hungry and became a comfort eater.

I feared returning to the poor little girl from the projects, so I worked as hard as possible and left little to no room for rest. Also, I feared becoming too much like my mother, so I became anxious about parenting my son the "right way."

"I was worried about being a good father. We'd never seen that; like never. There weren't very many examples for us growing up of that. We had like a high IQ for other things. I could tell you if somebody who walked into the room was plotting... But my emotional IQ was like minus 100 or so..."

-Jay-Z

So many of us are mentally fighting against ourselves!

The fight is sometimes quiet and subtle. We push away the desires of our heart because we aren't sure that we can truly ever have them, and we quiet our conscience because it often says the opposite of the louder message provided by society. We've been taught NOT to hear the wisdom of our soul and to long for external sources of relief.

I encourage you to ask yourself, *"What has happened, because of what happened?"*

What I've learned is that we aren't fighting simply because we want to; we are literally fighting for our lives and don't even know it! In our mind, emotional safety is just as important as our physical safety. Despite changing scenery or circumstances, traumatic memories (some that have even been passed down to us) stay with us throughout our lives consciously or unconsciously.

We are left constantly trying to rearrange the puzzle pieces of our lives, with little to no guidance on what the picture should look like. How many of our ancestors lived beyond survival? How many current examples do we have of emotionally healthy individuals that look like us?

Particularly, as Black people in America, we are impacted by psychological trauma at much higher rates. However, many of us are suffering in a silent sea of shame. An alarming number of us are born into environments that are not set up for us to thrive. Together, I believe we can reduce the stigma of mental illness by sharing our individual stories and supporting others through theirs.

According to the 2016 National Survey of Children's Health (NSCH), 45% of all American children have been impacted by Adverse Childhood Experiences (ACEs). However, the rate is nearly 20% higher among black, non-Hispanic children in the nearly all parts of the U.S.

All of these adverse experiences leave us with the challenging goal of undoing the multigenerational maladaptive behaviors and the correlating psychological impact as we navigate life with few or no healthy mentors to show us the way. Many researchers have found that these adverse experiences we face as children, often translates into toxic stress as our brains are still developing.

This stress actually changes the physical brain structure of a growing child and causes them to be much more vulnerable to irritability, anxiety, depression, suicide, substance abuse and unhealthy relationships throughout life.

Too often, we see mental health as one extreme or the other (healthy vs. "crazy"), rather than viewing psychological and emotional wellness on a spectrum. It's fluid and evolves. We become resilient when we learn how to express our emotions in healthy ways. The rule of thumb in our community has become, *"Don't feel and just move on."* We've been told that we *"don't have time to cry."* Then, when we get time, we fill it up by staying "busy," endeavoring to *give unto others...* but, to what extent?

I constantly ask myself, what's the REAL reason I feel such a deep longing to help others? If I'm honest, it is because I know what it's like to feel completely alone in the world, to be left, to feel invisible, to feel worthless, unwanted, anxious and scared. I became a therapist because I wanted to "help" anyone who looked like an earlier version of myself.

I see suffering, and it's very familiar to me. It's something I have an intimate connection with. I can relate deeply with the brokenhearted and discouraged, and I see a lot of hurt in our communities. This pains my heart since I know that the cycles are continuing. Too few of us who "made it out" are being honest about what we sacrificed in the process. We aren't sharing these critical stories! We only highlight the accomplishments, the success, and the "come up"; glazing over the trauma, the pain, and the horrific memories.

As you read this book, chapter by chapter, and story by story, you will be introduced to amazing people who have learned to truly own their story enough to help guide others through the very same process.

Hopefully, as you internalize these messages and reflect on how they can inspire you to become more in-tune with your own emotions, you will gain a deeper sense of how to accept them versus pushing them away. Perhaps you will dig a little deeper to consider if there are any parts of *your* story that are still tender.

My wish is that our stories will help you begin to think differently about mental health and emotional wellness. Regardless of the information you already have on the topic, reading these real-life experiences, might help you to visualize the complexities and benefits of the healing process.

You might find it helpful to keep a journal close by as you read each author's message, to take notes when something resonates with you. At times, you may feel sad, angry, or confused. Write about it and talk about it with someone who is trustworthy and emotionally safe. If you are anything like the person I was in 2015, you may not have access to many emotionally healthy & nurturing people in your life. Maybe you are surrounded by people who are *fighting* too. You may want to consider seeking unbiased and unconditional support from a licensed professional. Trust me, there really is no shortage! Over the last three years, I've somehow found over 20,000 of them.

The road might be long and hard. The work we do within our self is challenging; it may even be the most difficult thing you ever have to do. However, from where I'm sitting, I know personally and professionally that it's worth it in the end. I'm a witness and a firm believer of that.

I believe that we all experience our fair share of suffering in this world. Personally, I hope that my life (the good, the bad, and the ugly) is an example of all the possibilities available when we accept what has happened and honor the WHOLE story.

Each and every experience (and its related emotions) is meant to teach us something valuable about ourselves and the world around us. We don't always know where we are headed in this journey, and that's the most beautiful part. If we allow ourselves to remain open, we are bound to see the beauty of the process called "growth."

Paula Finn said it best:

"If you follow the desires of your heart, the integrity of your conscience, and the wisdom of your soul... then each step you take will lead you to discover more of who you really are, and it will be a step in the right direction."

And so, the journey continues...

YOUNG, DOPE, AND TIRED AF:

The Strengths & Struggles

of Black American Millennials

by Tiffany L. Reddick, LPC

My story isn't a hero's journey.

Well, it is, but it isn't. It is my story, and I do consider myself a superhero; like I do anyone whose chosen profession is saving lives. However, this isn't a typical hero's journey archetype where you will see me take on a clearly epic challenge, embark on a specific epic quest, suffer a definitive epic fail, recover precisely and (of course) epically, only to learn the true purpose of the epic adventure was to learn a particular epic and redemptive lesson.

Nope... this chapter is none of that.

There are no towering peaks or low-lying valleys on my journey. In fact, it's pretty regular. I guess that's kind of the problem. But now I'm getting ahead of myself, so I guess I'll just start talking, or writing, or whatever, and hope I arrive at a point where this all makes sense by the end.

PART I

I'm almost gifted.

I say that not to brag and not as hyperbole, but in the literal sense. Learning was always easy for me; from the beginning of my academic career. In the third grade, after taking some standardized test that would supposedly measure whatever standardized tests administered to third graders are designed to measure, I received a letter stating that due to my high performance on the verbal section, I was going to be given another test; this one to determine my appropriateness for the "gifted program."

I was pretty excited, and my parents were proud.

A couple of weeks later, I took this "gifted test," and four weeks after this, we received the results. I didn't make it in. This happened TWO MORE TIMES during my formative years; once again in the fifth grade, and then once more during middle school.

Seriously? Who puts a kid through this three times?

Just let me in the program, already! I can't say that I was crushed; however, I was disappointed, and by the third go-round, frustrated.

If I had to pinpoint a place in my life where my secret obsession with achievement began, this would probably be it; my earliest memory of feeling as if I was not good enough. Once you get an official letter stating you are almost gifted, you can't really go back. My parents, particularly my mother, would not have let me, even if I had wanted to.

The bar was set and locked in on high.

I was raised in a typical black, middle-class home. My parents— both brought up in working class, urban environments, and individually fueled by a desire to do something bigger with their lives than their current situation would likely allow—joined the military; where they met, courted, and a couple of assignments and one baby girl (yours truly) later, married.

Eventually, my two younger sisters joined our nuclear family, with my parents feeding the three of us messages that I imagine every black, middle-class parent (who sought to guarantee their children had all the opportunities they did not) fed their children. "Don't bring any C's in this house" and "Don't let me find out you are acting a fool in these white people's school" were common lectures.

Once, after I innocently told my mother I wanted to be a nurse, she replied, "Why? You are smart enough to be a doctor. Don't settle for less than what you are capable of."

Career aspiration immediately amended.

And it worked. I successfully advanced through high school, college, and even graduate school; riding on what I had no idea at the time were some of the most common symptoms of attention deficit hyperactivity disorder, including limitless energy, hyper-focus, and increased motivation up against impending deadlines.

Oh, and it didn't hurt that I was smart. Smart enough to use every trick in the book to overcompensate for my self-diagnosed "laziness" caused by my undiagnosed psychiatric disorder.

Looking back, I was actually just a conscientious student who recognized when to show up and pay attention, which assignments to skip versus torture myself over completing, when it made sense to change my major—after seeing how many math and science courses Pre-med required—and allowed myself to accept C's and D's in courses that "didn't matter."

If my school-aged "self" had been a current client, I would say "Oh, so you are playing to your strengths," or "I see you working smarter, not harder," and "You have to do what works to reach your goals, girl." But at the time, these tactics felt like cheating, underachieving, and selling myself short.

On really bad days they felt like failures.

In 2007, I graduated from the University of West Georgia with a Master's of Education degree in Guidance and Counseling, and a severe case of imposter syndrome. I was unable to accept the accomplishment as something I earned or deserved.

Like every other bright-eyed, bushy-tailed, millennial with a fresh degree and a crap ton of student loan debt, I was eager to change the world, make money, and be great. My cup runneth over with ambition, yet lacked strategy.

A combination not likely seen in a recipe for success.

I was a first-generation college graduate, and to my knowledge, no one in my family had reached this level of education; which means there was no blueprint. I hadn't formed a strong connection with any professors or supervisors. I can't put my finger on why not.

Maybe I was so focused on getting "it" done, everything else seemed unimportant. Maybe I was too busy; working full-time in school doesn't leave much time for finding and nurturing professional relationships that MIGHT lead to an underestimated advantage at an unknown future date.

Or, maybe it was the imposter syndrome, and I was scared of being discovered. Afraid my secret identity would be revealed, and everyone would learn that I was just... regular. And there is no place in this world for regular black girls.

At least not any place I wanted to be.

I knew there were women, my age, maybe even younger, who worked harder than me, overcame bigger odds than I did, got better grades than me, had bigger and better dreams for the programs they would create that would have better outcomes for their clients, and who, in 20 years, would get better awards.

These women probably—no, DEFINITELY—knew what they were doing, instead of furiously looking up counseling interventions minutes before sessions with my clients.

And they were more than likely able to complete the piles of necessary paperwork without stimulant medication and a shot of tequila. No, being almost-gifted was not going to cut it anymore. I was going to have to do something to get ahead of this. So, I leaned further into my young, fabulous, and unbothered persona to check promotions, degrees, and vacations off the to-do lists; uploading pictures as proof that I was anything but... *regular.*

Now, of course, my mother and several other well-meaning people explained the necessary steps to the sure path of turning an advanced degree into a nice stable life.

Yet, it didn't "feel" right.

Such a millennial thing to say, right?

Their suggestion of a respectable government or corporate gig did not seem like it would lead to changing lives on a grand scale, and honestly, they felt more like what I was trying to avoid, no escape—a life of settling and mediocrity—the hallmarks of "the regular." I wanted excitement, adventure, and experiences, all while creating preventative programming that positively shaped every young mind it touched and afforded me a comfortably luxurious lifestyle. Oh, and I wanted it NOW.

Not on some 20-year life plan.

Let me take a moment right here to shout out our parents' generation, the Baby Boomers. And specifically, my favorite Boomer, my Mama, who is quick to engage me in a discussion about my contribution to this book and what it means for my business and in the same breath, tell me to check my email for job openings at the Center for Disease Control she forwarded me.

Let's be real; it's the Boomer's sacrifices, sensibilities, and safety nets that have allowed many a millennial the privilege of following our hearts to chase our unrealistic dreams and expectations.

The ignorant 20-something that I was at the time believed these expectations made complete sense and seemed achievable in a couple of years. All my life, I was told that I could do anything. Every day, I read stories online of young millionaires and moguls, whose ideas were changing the way we live, worked, and played. This was around the time the Obamas happened, and every excuse seemed null and void.

If you didn't "make it," it had to be your own fault.

Spoiler Alert: I didn't 'make it.'

At least not according to how I defined success. At first, it looked and felt like I was doing pretty well. I was working in the field I had pursued my degree in, I owned a cute little townhouse, I had a solid group of friends, I was taking vacations, and had a little rotation of romantic interests. All of this in the Black Mecca that was - *is* - Metro Atlanta, Georgia.

I was living my best Black Sex in the City inspired life.

And you couldn't tell me *nothing*.

I wouldn't have listened to you anyway.

But, that was all surface. Underneath, I was a whole mess. Living paycheck-to-paycheck, I managed to two-step my way into the same traps they told me to go to school to avoid. While in my field of study, my first job out of grad school was not the $50-60k annual salary school counselor career I had hoped for, but a $30k a year community counseling job.

I had graduated, and the student loan refund checks stopped running. My ends stopped meeting and were more like awkward acquaintances waving at each other from a distance. I have money avoidant tendencies, and as the gravity of my financial situation brought me down on my ass, I just buried my head and became willfully ignorant. I was regularly robbing Peter to pay Paul.

To be fair, my base expenses would have likely been covered if not for a few bad habits that made for regularly occurring unexpected expenses.

Case in point: speeding. On average from about 2004- 2010 I averaged at least three moving violations and an accident a year. I also went out and ate and drank with friends fairly regularly in an attempt to distract myself from the hot mess that was my personal life. I was generally a poor planner with no budget to cover expected irregular expenses and my finances remained in a permanent caught-off-guard status, wreaking havoc on my already low self-esteem.

At one particularly low point, I ran out of gas on the way home from work. So ashamed, I sat in the car for hours bawling until my direct deposit hit, and I could call roadside assistance for the minimum seven dollars they charge for their gas delivery service.

In her bestselling book *Rising Strong*, shame researcher, Brené Brown, calls the barriers we put up to avoid reckoning with our true emotions, as *offloading hurt*.

Overachievement, procrastination, overcompensating, poor boundaries, perfectionism, detachment, numbing, comparison, and overspending all fall into this category of avoidance. The strangest part is if you had asked me if I was miserable. I would have honestly said no, I wasn't depressed, anxious, or angry. Most of the time, I was having a blast. These offloading strategies kept me comfortable for a little while.

Now, what I was feeling was exhaustion, overwhelmed, and increasingly uncertain that I was making the right choices in my career, that I had chosen the right career at all. These physical and mental symptoms are often the result of offloading hurt. But, as I looked around and commiserated with my friends at happy hours I probably couldn't afford to attend, I recognized most of us felt this way.

So, instead of looking deeper, I accepted this reality as the price I would have to pay to avoid being seen for what I thought I was... regular. I was afraid to admit I was wrong, that I was making mistakes in my work with clients. I couldn't afford my lifestyle, and I increasingly despised what I did for a living. I did not want to admit that 'adulting' was hard and I was struggling.

You can probably guess where this is going. Eventually, I hit a wall. I stopped working; I gave up the clients I was assigned and strongly considered leaving the field of mental health. I nearly turned my back on a career that the past five years of my life was dedicated to.

In twenty-something years, that's nearly a lifetime. I had to do something different; this way was killing me.

I wish I could say that there was one major turning point in this moment. That one epiphany, a particular therapy session, or a specific medication or strategy brought me out of this slump. If there was, I don't remember it. What I remember is a slow recognition that I had lost myself. Or maybe, I never really knew myself, never taking the time to explore what I wanted and how to pursue it. All the work I was doing to keep from being seen as... regular, I had hidden me, *the real me*, from myself.

Fortunately, the knowledge and experience I have in mental health helped me avoid a true crisis; yet, there were some close calls; a few days of literally dragging myself to my computer or cell phone and calling on the entire Holy Trinity, *and* Mary AND Martha for the grace of a few minutes of productivity. Occasionally, there were thoughts. I won't describe them as suicidal because they weren't, but these thoughts were dripping with so much hopelessness, my counselor's mind ignored all of the red flags they raised.

I began meditating.

And then, I began running, chanting affirmations of life, as my worn sneakers hit the pavement. I made sure I ate regularly, and as balanced a diet as I could afford, using my stimulant medication to inhibit appetite. These tactics, which I later learned are essential therapeutic lifestyle habits, worked, and slowly cleared a path of clarity, which cut through my brain fog. Ultimately, I decided, going forward, I would only pursue employment that involved work that I was eager to do and outlined what it would look like.

"I want to do a lot of the things I want to do, and none of the things, I don't," I told a friend. He laughed at my audacity and told me life doesn't work that way. Shortly after, I got a job that looked much like the description I typed into a blank Evernote just a month or two prior. It's only now, as I am going through the process of pulling this story from my memory into words on a page, that I recognize that my fear wasn't – *isn't* – that I am regular.

Or, even worse, that I am "basic," which is the millennial equivalent of the kiss of death.

Therefore, my actual fear is that I am not enough.

Not smart enough, accomplished enough, or *enough* enough. Somewhere in between explicit lectures and implicit bias, the idea my value as a person wasn't inherent, that it had to be earned, implanted itself in my subconscious and like some opportunistic weed takes every opportunity to sprout; snuffing out confidence and courage, replacing it with self-doubt and shame.

> *"I define shame as the intensely painful feeling or experience of believing that we are flawed and therefore unworthy of love and belonging."* -Brené Brown

Nevertheless, I didn't think I belonged in this book. After hearing a few co-authors stories, the hardships many of them had overcome, and the amazing ways they influence lives daily, I doubted my regular, degular, smegular story would inspire or impact anyone. It took me a long time to finish my contribution.

Several times I contemplated emailing our coordinator and withdrawing from the project. Maybe if I waited until Volume 2 was commissioned, I'd have gone through some things, suffering enough to provide something valuable to you, the reader.

Yeah, I know it sounds stupid *now*, as I'm typing it. Fortunately, self-awareness is my superpower; finely tuned by therapy and professional development. I was able to recognize my comparison to others, and urge to sink into the bushes of anonymity, Homer Simpson meme style, until I had "earned" my place. My shame had been triggered. I don't have a lot of space to get to the full description of things, but I will tell you the only way the feelings of unworthiness and inauthenticity will be defeated is with vulnerability, appropriate emotional exposure, uncertainty, and risk.

So, here I am.

My story is enough because I am enough; worthy of love and belonging. My humanity, as does yours, reader, deserves to be seen. As. Is. - from basic to #BlackExcellence - and every level in between.

I started by saying this isn't a hero's journey kind of story. I wished it came to some sort of victorious and final end. I imagine myself standing on the edge of a waterfall in the royal challenge scene in Black Panther, triumphantly accepting my place as queen after throwing my challenger over the edge.

But, that's not how any of this works. I continue to recommit to my process. Recommit to finding joy in progressing towards living in my whole humanity. Some days this is a daily ritual. Other times it's hourly. On bad days (yes, therapists have bad days too), I make it a moment by moment effort. These are the ugly moments you rarely see the 'Gram.

This is what therapy looks like once you are off the couch, out of the office, and back in reality of unsafe places. This is "the work." I am worth it. We are worth it.

You are worth it.

PART II

"Just because we are magic,
does not mean we aren't real."
-Jesse Williams

"WTF is wrong with me? I've been through way worse than this sh*t..." "Why is this happening now?" "Am I crazy? Am I going to have to be on meds the rest of my life? I can't do this right now; I have things to do, can this wait?"

I used to work as an admitting clinician in a psychiatric emergency room. When there was a concern that someone may be dangerous to themselves or others, they would end up sitting across from me. They would tell me their life story, and we worked together to figure out if this concern for their safety was strong enough to warrant a few nights stay in our stabilization unit. I assessed hundreds of people of all ages and walks of life. My favorites, for lack of a better word, were the overachievers.

In addition to having a strong reputation in the community, the facility had contracts with several prestigious colleges and universities and specialized in treating licensed professionals in recovery. We were frequently the first recommended on many employee assistance programs' lists.

So, included with my personal experience as a recovering perfectionist/overachiever, I've also got some professional experience in this game.

Have you ever watched a dramatic movie or television program where there is some horrific, tragic, incident, and a wounded person on a gurney comes to, learns what happened, and then begins fighting to get off the gurney? They are swinging on first responders, while desperately trying to return to the metaphorical—or, perhaps literal—train wreck that had rendered them unconscious just moments prior?

Yeah... that's how the overachievers, sitting on the couch in an assessment room of a psychiatric institution sounded, as they futilely attempted to bargain their way out of inpatient treatment. In my most therapeutic tone, I'd explain, "Ma'am/Sir, you are experiencing the mental health equivalent of taking a bullet through a vital organ. We cannot give you a Band-Aid and let you run back into a war zone."

We, the young and hungry, do a version of this every day. Eagerly climbing the socioeconomic ladder and attempting to make our families and ancestors proud, while collecting coins and making it all look easy for the culture, as our aspirational personas disregard the impact of our reality.

Wounded by daily racial and sexual aggression (macro and micro), vicarious traumas, and our lack of self-compassion and kindness, we self-diagnose the severity of our injuries and bandage our own injuries using achievement, technology, and boozy, bottomless brunches as an anesthetic.

Can we take a deeper look into this for a minute?

What's actually driving the #BlackExcellence "movement?" And where is it taking us? Why are we so willing to throw our wounded bodies back into the wreckage? The quick, dirty, and deeply unsatisfying answer: It's complicated.

We, the Millennials, were born in a remarkable time; a generation of firsts, and arguably one of the most heralded and hated. Personal computers became mainstream during our formative years. 9/11 occurred as we emerged into adulthood; forever altering our ideas of safety and privacy. Mobile phones, once only seen occasionally and mostly in cars (or Zack Morris' back pocket), have become indispensable.

The internet revolutionized the way the world does business, which resulted in sweeping change across industries; how we live, work and play will never be the same. We have been told, in one way or another, that anything is possible.

Self-esteem curriculum, movies, and music spoon feed this message. And through the internet, we have proof as hood-to-Hollywood stories, and viral, seemingly-overnight success, play out daily across our Instagram feeds and Facebook timelines.

Not only that but if I can also have an aromatherapy diffuser with a built-in Bluetooth speaker delivered to my door in an hour with next no delivery charge, you would have a hard time convincing me that anything is impossible.

Our speed of life has rapidly accelerated, and with it, our expectations of the world and ourselves.

And we are killin' it!

It is an AMAZING time to be young, black, and gifted. We are founding multi-million-dollar startups across industries.

We aren't just climbing the corporate ladder; we are dominating that bih. Glass ceiling, where? We are leading social change movements that are creating change. We are traveling all over the world and showing every corner the diversity and beauty of the diaspora. We are reclaiming our time while also spreading both #Blackgirlmagic and #Blackboyjoy.

There is now such a thing as trap yoga, y'all.

TRAP. YOGA.

We are outchea for real! We are leaving our big beautiful blackity black mark on the world, and we look FABULOUS while doing it. I know! I've seen our Instagrams!

Every day we LIT. Literally (no pun intended).

It's as if we have internalized every message preached on porches and the beauty salons and barber shops; from the church pulpit, the principal's office, and on the corners from dope boys who recognized we were one of the few who had what it takes to beat THE statistic.

You know the one.

I am the hope and the dream of the slave, indeed!

Yet, somehow, it is not enough.

There is more work. Always more work.

Thanks to our hyper-connected tendency, we have a permanent front row seat to the world's injustices that often disproportionately impact us, and those who look like us, in the worst ways. Feeling powerless, we watch them on our mobile devices, as we receive news of another black person who has suffered at the hands of those hired to serve as protectors.

We helplessly listen as family members or friends who didn't "make it," describe their challenges navigating the social services system; struggling to deal with them, as we desperately attempt to shake off microaggressions, before they take root in our psyche.

There is always another level.

Technology, particularly the internet, has equalized the playing field in many ways. It provides a digital link to almost anyone and anything; allowing us to level up—millennial speak for accomplishing a goal—faster than what was believed possible; however, the curse of that often-delivered gift is "social comparison."

Social comparison theory states that we determine our own social and personal worth based on how we stack up against others. Of course, social media did not create this phenomenon, but Facebook, Instagram Snapchat, etc., send it into overdrive.

"Mirror, Mirror in our hands, who is the fairest, dopest most successful, most well-traveled in the land?"

When the answer will inevitably be "not you, bih!" our ego, the hustler, goes into overdrive; using perfectionism, busyness, and overachievement as evidence we deserve to be here.

This self-sacrificial cycle is deceptive since it is often rewarded externally at the expense of our wellbeing. We manage this current pain, dissatisfaction, and exhaustion, all while trying to outrun, outpace, and outwork the past traumas and unhealthy belief systems instilled in us during our upbringings; where even the most well-intentioned, prepared, and educated parent or guardian would struggle not to pass down messages that deny our inherent worthiness:

"You have to work twice as hard..."
"Don't let these white folks see..."
"You better not get up there and embarrass me..."

Just being allowed to "be" in the world is a privilege black folks are rarely provided, especially in the United States, where many of our not-so-distant ancestors were assigned a value and sold. So, we hustle hard to prove our value to the world; racking up debt, strained relationships, health conditions, and secret "nervous breakdowns," alongside degrees, promotions, likes and follows.

This is what you are experiencing when nothing is wrong. In fact, things look good, but something ain't right. Shame causes us to outsource our hard-earned successes as a win in a cosmic lottery or an offering in return for ancestral favor. It's easy to believe that struggle will be our permanent state. It is easy to believe joy is for everyone else but us.

And so, we hustle on.

We rise and grind. We join team no-sleep. We declare ourselves the kingpin, a girl boss, and post about making money moves. We defer love; whittling romantic, platonic, and familial connection and true intimacy down to intense, but brief digital flings, orchestrated through rushed text messages. We move to our next power meeting with our big aviator sunnies that conveniently dim the energizing sunlight; oblivious to the fact that nature is showing out today.

We forget to breathe.

There may be a meal; there might be some exercise because #GymFlow, but there will definitely and indefinitely be work. There is no time to waste when you are working twice as hard to get one-fourth as far- accounting for the fact you may be black and a woman, or non-binary, or Muslim or belonging to any other intersectional group whose privileges are routinely questioned. When Trump is in office daily threatening our basic human rights. When there is so much to be done. When so many are depending on us.

If not now, when? If not us, *then who?*

Our intentions are noble, our schedules are full, but our minds and bodies are running, running... always running on empty. Then we burn out.

Slow mental, emotional, and sometimes physical shut down. Work is left undone, lives are left untouched, and a generation of dreams indefinitely deferred.

Enter Therapy and Therapists.

An Ounce of Prevention

We all knew that was coming, right?

Our deeply melanated skin is not an emotionally protective factor. We are incredible, but we are not invincible. Our lives are full and beautiful and resilient; yet, still require safeguards that sometimes go beyond wellness trends and self-administered self-care.

Do you want to know my favorite thing about participating in therapy, both as a client and as a counselor? At its core, therapy is a practice in the art of "being." It is an unbiased, objective, and sacred space where you do not have to "produce" anything to be of value. Your presence is a present, and the constant thoughts that are running in your head throughout the day have a place where they can stretch out, get comfortable, be fully examined, and if necessary... let go. In a world where everything is a constant rush, I found that a place where my progress is not timed, or specifically measured, incredibly freeing.

And, at times, terrifying. But, mostly freeing.

The counselors and therapists I have had throughout my life guided my examination of the things I needed and wanted; freeing myself from the expectations of family, friends, lovers, and society. They helped me ground my wildly unrealistic and draining aspirational identity of being equally effortless, yet tenacious. They helped me grieve, as I killed the notion that I could be both.

They facilitated my process of separating myself from my diagnosis and my reconciliation and acceptance of what I thought life would be... and how it actually turned out.

Therapy helped me recover from this classic millennial expectation hangover by mourning the loss associated with the difference in these two points. There can be a ton of grief work in counseling. It is worth the work.

Therapy helped me to acknowledge the toll my spirit was taking when I worked harder for less gain in all of the areas of my life, giving me a reprieve from the emotional labor of being the strong friend, the strong employee, the strong daughter, or the strong romantic partner. It allowed me to practice a different more-quiet-but-more-liberating strength.

The strength of vulnerability.

It helps me, yes. I currently have a therapist, confronting the fear of vulnerability as I move into the next chapter of my life; launching an online coaching and consulting practice.

But nothing was wrong, right?

Tuh.

As a high-functioning, high-achieving, generally healthy person who has proudly decided to use whatever privilege I hold to leave this world a better place, I think of therapy and therapists as personal trainers for our emotions, keeping us mentally and emotionally in shape; an asset in today's trying times.

Some people see their therapists as an assistant who helps them unpack, and properly put away all their emotional "junk" they've stuffed, hidden, and buried, sometimes for years. But for me, a [relatively] young, black, and purposeful professional helper who intentionally chooses to take on what others can't and/or won't, I view my therapists as assistants but instead of always unpacking, much of the time they help me to organize and pack this voluntary extra baggage most effectively.

And sometimes, they save a little space in the corner of their office for storage and safekeeping when I need to leave a few things behind for a while, to ensure I keep enough room in my life for my own joy.

PART III

For this portion of our chapter, I am supposed to inform you what to do next, now you have seen the light, and recognize that therapy and therapists aren't just for "the broken and broken-hearted." But being the young, savvy, creative, type 'A' achiever that you are, you probably know exactly what actions to take.

Hell, I am sure you've probably already visited your insurance company's website, done a search that includes the preferred demographic details of who you would want to work with, googled their names, checked out their website, and highlighted your top choices; organizing the information into a spreadsheet and setting the intention to start calling your top three tomorrow.

No, instead of giving another thing on the list to "achieve," I am going to advise you of the opposite. Take no action. Not just yet. Be still for a few moments. Take three or four deep breaths; allowing your belly to expand and your shoulders to drop. Let the words in this chapter, and any other you may have read, wash over you. Take note of which parts resonated or stuck with you... and which parts did not.

Don't judge or question these thoughts. Simply notice them as they drift through your mind. If recalling a particular passage causes you to react in any way, take note of this, without judgment. Sit in the uncertainty of this moment, even if only for five minutes. When you finish, pull out a journal and jot down your thoughts, feelings, and insights.

I took you through this exercise because choosing a therapist often appears as the easiest part of the process. This is especially true when you are seeking one for the purposes of emotional hygiene. It is easy to believe that because you are functioning well, you can treat your emotional health casually, like a car needing an oil change; pulling into the next quick lube place you can find.

Please do not do this!

Conscientious auto owners know that proper and professional maintenance is key to the optimal performance and longevity of their vehicle, and never let just any old body perform work on their vehicles, without proper vetting.

As conscientious owners of the most sophisticated machines on earth, we should hold ourselves to the same standard. I know you are still itching for concrete actions to take, a process for moving forward.

Don't worry; I got you!

Review the notes you took following the mindfulness exercise above. Do any themes stand out to you that you think you would like to learn more about or explore more deeply? Were you physically or emotionally reactive towards any ideas or topics?

Would you like to have a safe, sacred, and nonjudgmental space to freely air out the frustrations of being "the strong friend" without reciprocation when you need it?

Using these insights, write down 3-5 questions to ask a potential therapist. Now, take your expertly curated spreadsheet of insurance provider approved counselors. From here I want you to pull up the profiles of the therapists of your choosing on common online directories like **Therapy For Black Girls**, **Psychology Today**, or **Open Path Collective**. You may even need to check out their LinkedIn or Facebook Business Pages.

Many therapists now offer brief consultations to determine if you are a good fit to work together, but even if they do not, as you read their listings and websites, use those beautiful critical thinking and investigative skills to determine if they've already answered your question(s) in some way. Cross-check the list of topics that moved you, with their areas of experience, training and or expertise they have listed.

You might be asking, *"But what if they don't have an online presence?"* My short answer? Run!

Just kidding... kind of.

In my humble and possibly controversial opinion, any professional not having a web presence in the 21st century is a strong indicator this professional may not possess the cultural competence to understand and fully empathize with the influence of technology in every area of our lives, and how this, in turn, impacts our well-being.

If it can be avoided, I'd advise against working with someone with no digital footprint, unless you received a strong recommendation from someone you trust. Also, time is of the essence. You are a busy professional, and every moment spent learning basics you could have read on a simple website, are resources you could be spending connecting with a therapist whose starting point is not quite as far back.

> #ProTip: If you are a corporate rockstar or intrapreneur, do not forget to check if your employer offers an employee assistance program (EAP), or other corporate wellness initiatives, they often include 6-12 free sessions with a licensed mental health provider you choose from their pre-approved list.

> Confidentiality still stands, and they will not communicate with your employer. You will likely have fewer options, but if you are ballin' on a budget and need to bootstrap your wellness, EAP's are a good solution.

Alternatives

I often tell people, mental health and wellness is a full body job. Regularly processing our thoughts, feelings, and choices are only one part of optimal mental functioning. There are several steps we can take in nearly every other area of life that will allow us to get out of our heads and into fully enjoying the "best life" so many are claiming to live.

For instance, regular exercise has been shown to be more effective than medication in treating depression. Spending time in nature decreases anxiety and blood pressure while improving our sense of peace and feelings of connectedness.

Speaking of connection, just hugging for 30 seconds floods our body with oxytocin; a hormone responsible for warm and fuzzy feelings that combat feelings of loneliness and isolation.

These are just a few strategies referred to as therapeutic life-style changes that you can begin to implement on your own to your jumpstart your mental hygiene routine, without the help of a therapist that can have a major lasting impact.

I just need you to start.

Start now.

Nothing has to be wrong in order to begin purposefully protecting your mental and emotional wellbeing. You deserve to experience the same joy and light you bring to others in the world.

YOU are reason enough.

Okay, so I will admit my intentions have some self-serving motives. We do need you, and we need you at your best. This wild, wide world needs the change that you are fighting so fiercely to bring to it.

We need your cures, your companies, your activism, and your technologies. But, greater than that... we need *you*.

We need you whole, and able to fully, and deeply, appreciate the magic you create; the world-changing magic that you are.

BEHIND THE SMILE

by Khalilah A. Williams, MA, MFT

As a Marriage and Family Therapist, focused on disrupting dysfunctional relationships and stabilizing the family by encouraging them to adopt healthier patterns, I strive to understand the invisible rules of the family that dictates its function. With my support, individuals, couples, and families have identified how dynamics within their family can affect their psychological health, and they have developed the necessary skills to improve their lives.

It wasn't until my own experience as a Black woman struggling with the baby blues, feeling guilty and ashamed as a mother, and not having a safe place to explore my feelings that my passion for this topic came about. During this journey with me, I will help you identify the signs and symptoms of postpartum depression, identify resources for support, and develop the confidence to openly discuss your feelings and seek help.

*"Black people don't suffer from stuff like that;
we got way too many things to do besides worrying
about some postpartum depression."*

Those are the words that played in my head while I sat on my bed feeling overcome by emotions I was unaware that I had. I felt as if I was in a dark hole, spiraling with no end; it was pitch black, and I was wrestling with the idea that maybe I could have postpartum depression.

Yet, the feeling of shame would not allow me to accept it.

I was born in Jamaica around women who were considered to be strong by everyone; women who held it together when their lives were falling apart, and women who never allowed the world to see their imperfections.

Subconsciously, I was raised to associate natural emotions as weaknesses and failures. Being surrounded by women, who I viewed as being strong and the epitome of great motherhood, made me harder on myself. Unintentionally, I was creating a higher expectation of how I should perform in my new role. My concept of how things should be was shaped by the expectations of my values system. Some of which were unrealistic, which triggered anxiety in me, and I easily became irritated when things didn't go as planned.

As a 33-year-old new mother, with no idea of what the journey of motherhood would be like, or where it would take me, I did a lot of dreaming and planning for this special experience and the positive influence it would have on my life. I would now be responsible for the development and nurturing of someone else, the legacy that I will leave on this earth.

Therefore, I wanted to be equipped with the best skills and tools to be successful. I read books and blogs, watched programs, and of course, I googled just about everything.

I remember journaling daily about my experiences, beaming because I wasn't sick throughout my pregnancy, and able to partake in most activities as I had before. Things didn't go quite as I expected, and I struggled to bounce back when I was experienced emotional lows and feelings of unhappiness or distress. What I was experiencing was out of the norm for me because I'm usually able to overcome anything thrown my way.

Not being able to control the sadness and the irritability I felt produced great frustration with myself.

After having the baby, my mother stayed with my husband and me for the first week, and then my husband took a week off from work to help with the baby. Following those first two weeks, I felt alone, as if everyone had left me.

It was like I woke up one morning and everyone was gone.

Daily, I gave myself pep talks and fought back the tears; tears that I did not understand. Every day I told myself that I would feel better and that things would just fall into place.

No, I can't cry, I have things to do. This is a moment of weakness, and I can't allow it to happen. My energy was low, and my anxiety was through the roof. I worried about everything: *Was the baby eating enough? Was I pumping enough milk? Was the house clean enough?* The list went on and on and on.

Soon, I became an expert at willing my tears away.

I remembered thinking about my pregnancy and how amazing it had been; how prepared I was, and now this... how can I feel this way? What happened to all the bliss and the "I woke up like this" moments?

All around me, I saw what I thought were perfect mothers; they seemed to have mastered the art of looking and feeling good. This made me question myself many times about my inability to hold it together, and most of all, my failing abilities as a mother. I was used to feeling confident most of the time, and this struggle was a blow to my esteem. Added to what I thought were my short-comings as a mother, I had to deal with feelings of not meeting the societal norms of motherhood.

Our beliefs are influenced by our communities, the media, friends, and family. These influences sometimes have a strong impact on how we see ourselves. At times, I found it difficult to listen to my own ideas of what motherhood should be. Though I knew there would be sleepless nights; I had dreamed of waking up daily with high energy to play with the baby.

I envisioned lots of day trips, taking funny pictures, playing dress up while still having time to enjoy the things I loved.

Breastfeeding for the first year was a goal of mine, and when my body no longer produced milk after three months, my self-esteem took another blow. Social media only increased my fretfulness; I felt as though all the mothers I saw were well put to-gether and seemed to be handling the challenges of motherhood with ease. Showers became the highlight of my day, and I found solace in the bathroom, where the warmth of the shower and having solitude brought me peace.

To make matters worse, I suffered from postpartum hair loss; my hairline receded, and I had to shave my entire head.

Of course, this affected my self-esteem as well, and I felt like someone was playing a horrible joke on me. I was ready for it to end. My husband tried his best to comfort me and provide me with some "me" time while working a full-time job, and my mother would encourage me to visit her with the baby and get some fresh air. This would work great... until I was left by myself.

Having others around me made things better for me because they would help me with the baby and allowed me time to myself to relax. Also, having adult conversations allowed me to connect with others and step away from completely focusing on the demands of motherhood. I felt like I was connecting with the world whenever I had visitors or visited with others; yet, I felt isolated and agitated when I was left home alone with my newborn.

For the first two or three months after delivery, I mostly stayed inside my home due to fear that my infant would get sick from germs in the environment and other people.

Getting out for a few minutes a day could have improved my mood because sunlight increases the "feel-good" mood hormones in our body. I was thinking of the health and safety of my daughter. However, I wasn't considering the impact that isolating myself would have on my mental health.

Several months after giving birth, I visited my grandfather's gravesite. It was a cold afternoon; the air was crisp, and the earth was frozen. For some unknown reason, all of the tears I had held back came rushing out of me like a flood. I just sat on the ground and cried.

I wept alone, in a cemetery surrounded by dead people, which was a representation of how isolated and empty I felt.

The cry felt good. It was like a weight had been lifted off my shoulders. I was finally able to cry, knowing that there was no one around to judge me for not being what I perceived as perfect. I realized that it was okay to admit that my new role was challenging and that sometimes I needed space—my own time—to do something for me… something that I enjoy. I had been so focused on my role of being a mother that I neglected to nurture myself while adjusting to the new role.

After this breakthrough, I began to explore the need to grieve the mother I fantasized about being and accepting the mother that I was. I also began contemplating the possibility of having postpartum depression and what it would mean for my family and me. This allowed me to begin pushing for a change because I wanted to heal. I knew this would take time, and I needed to start advocating for myself. However, I needed to be honest with myself. I was not Superwoman; I could not do everything by myself.

I started my healing by having a conversation with my husband about how I was feeling and what I needed from him. He looked at me with the saddest eyes that seemed to turn to irritation because he couldn't understand why I had kept this from him. Quickly, I realized that I had not actually asked for help, and I was in agony due to the pressure of having to do everything myself.

Then, I spoke to my mother about my experience, and she revealed to me that she too had battled with symptoms of postpartum depression. She shared with me the impact it had on her life and her understanding of how I may have felt.

Sharing my experience with others enlarged my support system. It was an eye-opener to the many challenges mothers experience, it allowed me to develop a sense of awareness of what my needs are and how to get my needs met. Through support from family and allowing them to help me, I began to slowly pull myself together.

Even when I felt like I didn't want to do something for myself, I pushed through and took advantage of the self-care techniques and resources that were available to me. I began journaling again which allowed me to release a lot of the emotions I was feeling.

Journaling also facilitated the organizing of my thoughts and creating more of a detailed plan for my days. I treated myself throughout the week to something I enjoyed; this included getting my nails done, going out for a milkshake, creating a playlist for the walks I began to take and allowing myself to take leisure naps.

You know that old saying, "when the baby sleeps, you sleep"? I began to apply that to parts of my days. This made me feel more rested, and my tasks didn't seem as hard as they did before. By incorporating these strategies into my days, I was forced to create a routine which benefitted my family and me in maintaining my sanity.

I found online parenting groups that provided me with helpful tips on parenting and self-care. Allowing people to help me and asking for help when I needed it relieved a lot of the stress I was experiencing. Speaking with others made me realize that I wasn't alone and that I should not feel ashamed or guilty about experiencing something I had no control over.

Having self-care moments became important to me because they helped me to feel rejuvenated when caring for my daughter. I had suffered in silence when I didn't have to.

Shame and fear had prevented me from communicating my feelings and experiences with loved ones. This could have fostered positive social contact, which then would have aided in relieving the stress I was experiencing. I had unrealistic expectations of motherhood, and when I fell short of meeting these expectations, I was embarrassed by what I thought was me failing as a mother.

Some of my anticipation of motherhood included the baby making me feel complete, being happy all the time, balancing who I am and caring for my family effortlessly. Focusing in on these idealistic views prevented me from being in the moment and enjoying my small blessings daily.

When I returned to work after eight months due to my maternal leave and shoulder surgery, I re-evaluated how I treated my female patients. I began to take a closer look at the different symptoms these women could be exhibiting in relation to postpartum depression.

Postpartum depression can be a source of maladaptive parental behaviors such as harsh punishment, verbal abuse and spending very little time with their children. Some of the women referred to me for treatments are either fighting to regain custody of their children or require support with developing and maintaining a healthy, secure attachment with their children. Their ability to be nurturing may be impaired, which can result in them becoming less responsive to their children's needs.

Children born to women who are experiencing postpartum depression can be irritable and hard to soothe, increasing the chance of that child being neglected. This creates an unstable attachment between the mother and child because the mother is more impatient and distant with the child. From my experience of working with mothers, postpartum depression may go untreated in mothers from low-income and minority families because of lack of access to resources and denial of their symptoms due to stigma and cultural beliefs.

Studies have shown that African American women are less likely to seek support or help for postpartum depression even though the risk is twice as great for this demographic.

When diagnosed, they are also less likely to follow up with treatment. The negative connotation associated with mental illness is one of the many reasons these women shy away from acknowledging their symptoms and seeking treatment. They internalize their symptoms and see them as shortcomings instead of looking for a way to improve their well-being.

Additionally, many women fear losing custody of their child or children because they believe that they would be labeled as unfit to care for them. Sometimes, it may be difficult for mothers to consider postpartum depression because they are comparing their symptoms to severe diagnoses with dire consequences. There are also myths that prevent women from seeking treatment such as "it is your fault" and "it will go away on its own."

However, postpartum depression is not something one chooses, and it should be treated by a professional. The goal of therapy is to equip you with the tools necessary to live a healthier quality of life by better managing the symptoms and underlying causes of postpartum depression. Therapy will provide you with an unbiased and safe space where you can express yourself without insecurities, guilt or shame.

Postpartum depression has been compared to feeling as though you're drowning but seeing everyone around you breathing. During those panicky moments, you're asking yourself, "Why am I not as adequate as other mothers? "Why am I so sad and hopeless?" "How do I turn my brain off or slow it down?" "When will I return to my old self and stop feeling so overwhelmed and start sleeping again?"

Though you may feel like you are the only person in the world experiencing this, and that no one will ever understand; you are not alone. Most new mothers experience the baby blues, which have similar symptoms as postpartum depression: irritability, anxiety, sadness, and fatigue.

The difference between the two is that the symptoms of the baby blues are milder than postpartum depression, and they last for about two weeks.

Some women who experience the baby blues go on to develop postpartum depression, which includes symptoms of fear, loss of appetite, excessive crying, and reduced interest. These symptoms can begin six months following delivery and last up to a year after giving birth. Other symptoms include withdrawing from friends and family, difficulty concentrating, headaches, and feeling weak.

Some factors can increase a woman's risk of postpartum depression such as: anxiety, increase in stress, sleep deprivation, and a history of depression.

Participating in therapy is an effective treatment for postpartum depression. In rare circumstances, some women go on to develop postpartum psychosis which is considered a psychological emergency. These symptoms are intense, and patients display paranoia, hallucination, confusion and extreme irritability.

Some women may attempt to harm themselves or the baby. In these instances, these women should not be left alone, and immediate care should be sought from a healthcare professional.

If you have experienced any of these symptoms, they are not a reflection of who you are; they are caused by the shift in the hormones in your body following birth.

In the work that I do, I empower women to recognize and change their negative thoughts and behaviors. Women begin to develop coping strategies to manage their feelings of distress effectively. I also support women, as they grieve the mother they thought they would be and embrace the mother that they are. At times, there may be a loss of self, and with the changes in your body and in relationships you once had, your self-esteem may also be affected.

During therapy, these struggles are addressed, and you will be able to not only cope with different symptoms you are experiencing but also build stronger relationships and support systems while increasing your confidence.

Inviting family members, friends, or whoever you consider support into therapy sessions is also important for your recovery. This allows you to ask for the support you need from them and address the changes in the dynamics of your relationships. This is also an opportunity for your loved ones to become educated on your experiences and learn ways to support you as you improve your overall wellness.

With involvement in therapy, over time, you will be able to learn and correct the false beliefs that you have held which contributed to postpartum depression. The many symptoms you have will become manageable because you will learn how to take them apart and gain the tools necessary to better cope with them.

You will begin to map out a healthier lifestyle and develop the structure essential to building the woman you would like to be.

Your feelings and experiences will be validated, and you will be connected to resources that will provide you with the support needed to successfully move forward. I believe that it is important that you identify the influences in your life that define what a mother looks like because this will allow you to understand the pressure that you place on yourself as a mother.

As someone who struggled with the baby blues, I remember internalizing everything I felt, saw and heard. The guilt and shame that I felt prevented me from asking for help and sharing how I was feeling with my loved ones. Hindsight is truly 20/20 because now I know I did not have to suffer alone.

I could have drawn on the support of the people around me which could have alleviated the distress I was experiencing. Sometimes, it may be hard for you to reach out to others for support because you may feel ashamed and fear judgment; but, suffering in silence only makes things more difficult on you, and puts a strain on your relationship with your loved ones.

Therefore, to support yourself as you adjust to motherhood, I recommend that you become more aware of your sleep patterns, appetite, thoughts and your mood. Being aware of these things can give you some insight into the support that you need. I also encourage you to speak about what you're experiencing with a family member or a friend that makes you feel safe.

Being surrounded by people who support you allows the transition to be easier, and your confidence in the role of a mother to be stronger. Knowing that you are not alone in your experiences is therapeutic in itself because it alleviates some of the pressure that you may place on yourself. Postpartum depression can happen to anyone; it does not discriminate.

To the family and friends who observe the changes in their loved ones, do not assume that things will get better on its own. Encourage her to speak with a medical professional about her experiences while letting her know that she is not alone. Find out from her what support she needs and provide her with it.

Still, mothers might be reluctant to accept the support because they may feel ashamed or uncomfortable allowing themselves to receive the help they need. Assist her with daily chores, especially caring for the baby and offering emotional support to her. Encourage outdoor activities during the day because exposure to a few minutes of sunlight daily can improve her mood.

There are two forms of treatment used to treat postpartum depression: psychotherapy and antidepressant medications. The choice of which to use is based on the severity of postpartum depression the woman is experiencing:

- Antidepressants are medications prescribed to balance out your mood. If a woman is breastfeeding, she should speak to her physician before taking any medication to ensure the safety of the baby.

- In psychotherapy, several types of treatment can be used to treat postpartum depression such as Cognitive Behavioral Therapy, Dialectical Behavioral Therapy, Eye Movement Desensitization and Reprocessing, Emotion-Focused Therapy, Couples Counseling and Interpersonal Therapy.

There are countless benefits for treating postpartum depression with psychotherapy; the impacted mother will learn coping skills that can be used for long-term and improve her quality of life. She will gain a better understanding of what is happening to her and be able to educate the people in her life on her experiences. Therapy will provide her with a safe place to explore her experiences and validate what she is feeling.

The positive changes that occur with the mother will create a better prognosis for the entire family system.

I have used a combination of these psychotherapy treatments with mothers that I have worked with in an effort to help them create and maintain boundaries in their relationships so that they can get the support and understanding that they need.

Another part of treatment is also ensuring that they get the needed support to identify and change beliefs and expectations and acknowledge underlying emotions that are causing their depressive mood. I promote self-care to the mothers I work with and use five self-care strategies that will support positive change and lessen depressive mood.

These strategies are:

1. Maintaining a healthy diet
2. Getting enough sleep and rest
3. Finding or reconnecting with past hobbies
4. Maintaining social support
5. And pampering yourself.

I recommend support groups or meetup groups to my clients as a form of social support; this allows them to connect with other women who may have similar experiences as they do and gain an understanding that they are not alone.

The importance of self-care should not be overlooked because it not only allows you to handle the stressors more effectively, but it will also boost how you feel about yourself. Improvement in how you feel about yourself can make you less vulnerable to feelings of hopelessness.

There is a stigma attached to mental health and mothers feeling the pressure of making everyone in their lives besides themselves a priority. Combined with feelings of denial, shame, fear, and guilt, this will prevent her from seeking the necessary support. If you or a loved one is experiencing symptoms of postpartum depression, do not wait to seek treatment in hopes that the symptoms will pass.

The earlier it's treated, the quicker the recovery. Waiting to treat the symptoms only will worsen your condition. Women can recover from postpartum depression and thrive in their lives. Your feelings are valid; be proactive in seeking treatment. Some helpful resources for postpartum depression include online forums such as *Postpartum Support International* online meetings (PSI) and *What to Expect* postpartum depression forums (whattoexpect.com).

PSI provides online resources for mothers, families, and professionals seeking information and support. This online resource provides free live telephone sessions weekly with an expert for mothers and fathers. These telephone sessions can be anonymous and serve as a platform for information and responses to your questions and concerns.

Also, the online *National Women's Health* information center (womenshealth.gov) provides insight into the struggle a woman and her family may encounter after she has a baby, along with telephone numbers to contact for further support.

Your local hospital and clinic are available to provide you with consultations and referral resources. Most county mental health departments should be able to assist women who are uninsured or underinsured in finding resources and providers.

Through my experience of working with mothers and struggling to balance self-care and motherhood, I have created the movement called "Mommy Take off Your Cape" to promote self-care to mothers. With my support, psycho-education, and empowerment, women begin to give themselves permission to care for themselves without guilt or shame. This increases their self-esteem and development of more effective parenting skills as they balance the many roles they have more efficiently.

After becoming a mother, a woman goes through physical and emotional changes which may be overwhelming for her; this may cause her to focus on others and neglect her own needs. In finding the balance between taking care of yourself and your role as a mother, I encourage you to focus on three things:

1. Redefining your independence
2. Identifying your priorities
3. Appreciating your alone time.

The truth of the matter is that we can be our best in the many roles we have if we take care of ourselves.

Self-care isn't selfish... it's protecting your well-being.

BRAND NEW ME:

The Power in Healing

By Chautè Thompson, LMHC

"There is nothing more rare, nor more beautiful, than a woman being unapologetically herself; comfortable in her perfect imperfection. To me, that is the true essence of beauty."

-Steve Maraboli

Butterflies are beautiful creatures, but nobody would say that the process they endured to move from what they were, to what they would become, was anything close to attractive.

Metamorphosis is a change of the form into a completely different one, the transformation from an immature form to an adult form. This happens to caterpillars as they become beautiful butterflies, but it also happens to us as we heal and transform into our new selves.

Experiencing emotional abuse, a failed marriage, the pain of not feeling valued in my relationship, and the emotional loss of my living father ignited a passion within me to heal and to experience what beautiful relationships are made of.

Healing is a process, and when you understand this process, you will be better equipped to walk confidently in your journey.

Many of us have experienced broken relationships, have felt unworthy and not valued, have lost loved ones to death or life changes and have struggled to make sense of the rollercoaster of emotions. Whitney Houston sings "Where Do Broken Hearts Go," and although she sings about a love lost, I can relate this to the broken heart from a father, who was physically present, yet emotionally absent. Meaning, I grew up with my father but was not blessed with the close-knit relationship I yearned for.

My parents separated for the first time when I was twelve, and I have never forgotten my father calling my siblings and me into the room and saying, "Your mother and I are not going to live together. Who do you want to live with?"

This question was devastating for me because I felt bad for my choice of wanting to live with my mother, knowing I valued both of my parents.

Visiting my father was not something I looked forward to because it wasn't actual time spent with my father but rather simply time spent at his house. When I think of a father-daughter relationship, I picture outings as a girl, dates as a teenager, random conversations, laughs, check-ins, and constant protection for "baby girl." This relationship should introduce a daughter to what she should expect from her man when she gets older. *Fairytale living* is what I call it, probably my defense mechanism.

However, as I've gotten older, I have begun to understand that although I have seen this relationship between some fathers and their daughters, it isn't something every daughter receives.

My parents decided to get back together, yet separated and divorced a second time when I was sixteen. Again, visitation was not relationship building. It was me in an empty room, listening to the radio, and my father in his room watching television.

After getting married, I finally decided to have a heart-to-heart with my father. I shared with him the longing for a close relationship with him.

His response?

...that *he is who he is*.

Needless to say, the relationship never grew, and in retrospect, I acknowledge that culture played its role in my father's relationship building techniques. Over the years, I've also realized that this longing has carried over into my current relationship.

I married my best friend!

While loving him, in hindsight, I was losing myself. I constantly tried to please him, and when I was failing, I found fault with myself and tried harder. I went through numerous seasons of transition; such as, marrying right out of college, getting pregnant during my first year of marriage, and starting grad school with a newborn while working full time and having my second child two years later.

In the midst of these changes, I worked hard to maintain a healthy relationship with my best friend, but all of my efforts to maintain, build, create, an intimate relationship with my husband were unsuccessful.

Yes, transitions are a part of life and relationships are beautiful. Still, I was dying emotionally as I yearned for attention from (and to be desired by) the man that I deemed my other half. The emotional disconnect I had received from my father ended up being the same disconnect I received in my marriage.

Years into my marriage, I was made to feel like moving from a size 3 to a size 6 was unacceptable and undesirable; being human was frowned upon, and I was not valued. Every conversation I wanted to have for clarification or sharing my heart was met with anger, frustration, miscommunication, and the silent treatment.

I lost my voice in my relationship as we walked on eggshells, and he threatened divorce or spoke of his indecisiveness of wanting to remain in the relationship. I was fearful of losing the individual I deemed my other half.

In addition to this, my husband was taking numerous trips annually to another country with his friends or solo knowing I was not fond of the relationships he developed while away. This distance fueled my feelings of not being valued and my voice not seeming to matter in the relationship. Dealing with this for years in my marriage led me to finally stand up for me!

Although there are numerous ways to move through the healing and transformation process, for me, several things supported me on my journey; specifically, scripture, music, poetry, an understanding of how to move through the grieving process, self-care, and therapy.

I will also recommend a few others; however, know that you can tweak as necessary and add your own spin to make it work for you.

SCRIPTURE:

Matthew 6:33 informed me that I need to seek God and all His righteousness, and it brought me back to my foundation. For me to truly be at peace with losing my best friend and transition into being a single mother, I needed to seek God first. When I did that, my focus was shifted to being faithful and the reminder that God WILL take care of me—ALL of me—physically, mentally, spiritually, and EMOTIONALLY!

Psalms 139:14 reminded me that I was fearfully and wonderfully made. This, for me, was powerful because I did not feel beautiful to the one individual I wanted to be beautiful to - my husband. Seeing in the Bible that I am made beautiful, wonderful and worthy of more than I was receiving motivated me to see myself as more, carry myself as more and believe I was more.

Talk about the transition of a mindset shift!

Psalms 138:8 shared with me the Lord will perfect that which concerns me. This was life-changing for me because it meant God was dealing with my pain, my hurt, my shame, my sadness, my disappointment and my fears. God was carrying me through my healing process.

Each of these texts, along with a prayer life and blessing of a support system carried me through the healing process.

MUSIC

Songs and poetry tell life-stories, and when we find one that becomes our mantra, it is life changing! The one that was for me was Alicia Keys' "Brand New Me." It sang to my heart, empowered me, and now motivates me as I continue to see my GROWTH! As I listen to "Brand New Me," I was reminded that throughout my relationship I lost myself and when I started therapy, I found my voice. I began to speak up, and I became more confident in taking the steps that were needed to be a better version of myself. I found the courage to live; even if that meant without the person I deemed my best friend.

As I listened to this song, I moved from tears to smiles.

I am a completely different person now! I am empowered by this song knowing every word she sang was my life and is the individual I have grown into.

POETRY

Since poetry helps me to heal, I wrote poems to process and heal. To begin with, my emotions were EVERYWHERE!

Therefore, *Hibernate* and *Let Go* were written at two different stages of my healing process.

Hibernate was written at the beginning stage of my healing, a couple of months after my divorce. This poem speaks about the emotional turmoil I endured, and it speaks of being in a room full of people yet still feeling alone. It also speaks of the days people ask, "How are you?" and we say a simple "okay," knowing we want to scream *"far from ok, I'm dying inside."* Yet, we know a simple "okay" is all we can manage to get out of our mouth.

This poem speaks to the fear of allowing oneself to feel again, the risk involved and the desire to stand back and wait. It remains hopeful even though the emotion involved is overwhelming, and it ends with the hope of a happily ever after while sitting in the wisdom that *emotionally*, now is not the right time for any of that.

HIBERNATE
By: Chautè Thompson

Drowning in emotions
Gasping for air
Fighting for my life
Dying...

Giving life to new beginnings
As I struggle to understand
How this new me
Interacts with the old

Masking the pain
Smiling in the rain
Receiving band-aides
When surgery is necessary

Roller coaster of emotion
Curves, dips, highs, lows
Experiencing the rush..
What goes up... Must...
Scared to crash!

Don't want to be burned
Taking it slow

Winter arrived...
Hibernation

Looking forward to spring
Expectations...
Uncertain outcomes...
Until then...
Hibernate!

Let Go was written during the acceptance stage of my healing. This poem speaks to the facts of what is *no more,* moving into forgiveness, acceptance, and a new mindset.

LET GO:
By: Chautè Thompson

It's time to let go
Let go of the pain
Let go of the dream
Let go of the fact that we'll never be

Let go of if things were different
Let go of what was...

Let go

Now, the process might look different for you but know that having healthy distractions such as hobbies, spending time with loved ones, and finding creative ways to express yourself contributes to your healing.

It is imperative that you spend time understanding what it is that you are feeling and making sense of it, so it's not bottled up inside leading to anxiety and depression, on top of numerous other mental and physical health concerns.

5 STAGES OF GRIEF

We grieve when we lose a loved one to death, but we also grieve when we lose relationships or when situations in our lives change. Going through heartbreak raises numerous questions within yourself. The self-doubt is heightened, and the anger or resentment is also at its peak.

There's a process of grieving which must be experienced before healing can take its course.

There are five stages of grief; it is natural to move between them as there is no order to experience them. These stages are denial, anger, bargaining, depression, and acceptance.

DENIAL: As stated in my eBook *Everyday Survival as a Divorcée*, denial helps us to survive; it helps us to cope. During this stage, our body is only allowing us to feel what we can handle. Once you start to accept the reality of the loss and start to ask yourself questions, you are unconsciously beginning the healing process. The denial will begin to fade, and you will become stronger as the feelings you denied surface.

ANGER: The second stage is anger which is a necessary stage of healing. When you allow yourself to feel the anger, it will eventually dissipate, and healing can occur. We have primary and secondary emotions: primary is the anger; it's the first emotion, which is easier to feel than taking the time to know the true cause of our pain. Secondary emotions are the true emotions: disappointment, sadness, shame, etc. As you start to heal, you will pay more attention to the true emotions, and the anger will decrease.

BARGAINING: During this stage, you are thinking, processing, and speaking to God or your higher power about how the outcome can be different. You are attempting to negotiate your way to different outcomes, the "what if" and "if only" statements, considering what we could have done differently.

DEPRESSION: In this stage of the grieving process, you are overwhelmed with sadness. It is important to remember that it is natural to feel sadness from a loss. During this depression, you might withdraw, isolate yourself, and feel uninterested in events or things you once enjoyed. You might be able to get through your days with a smile, but once you get home, you are detached from the world.

ACCEPTANCE: The last stage is acceptance. Acceptance does not mean you are okay with the loss per se; it means you have accepted the reality of the facts. You learn to live, re-adjust as necessary, and move forward without this individual in your life.

A breakup ignites a roller coaster of emotions in addition to the fear of starting over! You might be asking the "what if" questions, determining if your choices and behaviors were the best, playing out scenarios in your head of moments in your relationship, and trying to figure out how it could have been different. You might be angry at the facts of yesterday while sitting in the reality of now and being fearful and unsure of how to move forward.

So, what did the stages of grief look like for me?

Well, sadness overwhelmed me. I took care of others throughout the day and was numb at nights. I was hurt that I had given my all to my marriage and fought long and hard for my relationship, but I still felt as if all my fighting was not good enough. I played so many scenarios in my head of what I could have done differently and would any of it change the choices my husband chose to take.

I even questioned if I could live with those emotions of not being valued in order to stay in the relationship. I battled with what was best, as I believed my children deserved to see what a warm, loving home looked like, instead of husband and wife living like roommates.

Also, I struggled with building my relationship with God. I was depressed, and I didn't want to pray. I didn't want to think. I didn't want to put effort into anything.

Moving from sadness to acceptance takes an extra effort. The more reality sets in, the more sadness becomes evident.

However, as I processed and moved between the stages, I was able to reflect on my experiences and transition into a healthier mindset, accepting myself, my experiences and my growth. I wrote poetry, went to therapy, made use of my support system and focused more and more on ME.

The foundational relationship that I had with God kept me, in addition to the scriptures that gave me comfort and hope. I also spent time painting, which proved therapeutic. There wasn't a care in the world that I focused on when I painted.

I hated to hear the statement "time heals all wounds" as I wanted the time to be now, but I can honestly say that as time passes and processing occurs, the pain does diminish.

Although reality remains reality, the ability to live, create a new norm, and form new traditions enables us to evolve and grow into better versions of ourselves.

RECOMMENDATIONS

1. Practice Self-Care

"Self-care is not selfish.
You cannot serve from an empty vessel."
-Eleanor Brown

As you are rediscovering yourself, spend some time in self-care/self-love. When you are moving from pain to the journey of rediscovering yourself, it is important to go back to the basics: Who were you before this relationship? What "likes" have you put on a back burner because you were nurturing your relationship? What do you currently want to try that you haven't tried before?

Date yourself!

During this time, I wrote my '40 before 40' list. It was exciting to find things that I had never done before, and I started venturing out to do them. It was also amazing how much I learned about myself, as I took steps to do what I enjoyed or to meet goals I had never thought to attempt in the past. My list included adventure, financial goals, family time goals, future purchases I wanted to work towards, travel plans and more!

2. Journaling

Another recommendation I would share is journaling.

I know that as you hear "journaling," you might cringe or skip over that word because it's mentioned all the time, but let's be creative. Journaling helps you to process your emotions, make sense of the emotions, and come up with ways to better understand, which all aid in helping you to cope. Without journaling, the feelings are bottled up, and the sadness, anger, frustration, or pain is not being released.

There's more than one way to journal: there's the traditional journaling of pen to paper, there's video journaling, where you keep a video diary, and there's a picture collage journal where you can collect memes, pictures, and quotes that express how you currently feel... and how you hope to feel.

3. Book Suggestions

My next recommendation is that you read *Sometimes you Win, Sometimes You Learn* by John Maxwell. This book sets the stage that life does not always go the way you intend. Although Maxwell's book focuses more on goals, it can give much value to those of us who have experienced a loss in our relationship.

It's easy to feel like a failure throughout the process, but it is imperative that the experience is looked upon as a learning experience. What have you learned about yourself, your desires and your interactions? How has your behavior played a role in the breakup, and how can you be stronger and better for your next relationship or even your singleness?

Another book suggestion is Gary Chapman's *The 5 Love Languages*. This book will help you to more clearly recognize your needs and the needs of your loved ones (children & anyone you date or marry). By better understanding your needs and the needs of your loved ones, you can be more aware of how love is portrayed.

An additional book suggestion is Alexandra H. Solomon's *Loving Bravely*. This is a good book to delve into before you place yourself back on the market. It teaches you 20 lessons to self-discovery and helping you better understand yourself, your family dynamics, and the role it plays in your mate selection, which opens your eyes to new perspectives and beautiful ways to interact with yourself and others.

4. Therapy

Although this is the last recommendation, it is certainly not the least. Therapy is God-sent! I recommend that it be used with each of the recommendations above.

Therapy provides a safe space to truly speak your heart without judgment, to talk through the "what-ifs" and to break down irrational thoughts. This enables you to challenge perspectives through non-confrontational approaches while working at your own pace and discussing topics which are dear to your own heart. Therapy helps you to make sense of the experience, learn ways to cope, and understand your behaviors so that you can grow in total acceptance of yourself. Overall, it will help you to embrace your truth and have the ability to move forward unapologetically.

Finding a therapist requires some effort. To start, search the internet for counselors in your area. Find someone who you perceive as warm and inviting. Look over their biography, their website, call them and take advantage of the 15-minute free consultation so you can get a better feel if this person might be a good fit. Ask the therapist about their specialty areas.

Work with a therapist who specializes in transitions, relationships, or grief. These are all areas that might deem helpful for you. Most importantly, if you choose a counselor but you feel it isn't a good fit, ask for recommendations to another therapist or search again.

For myself, I moved from being scared to express myself in my relationship because I did not want to upset my husband and endure threats of divorce, to finally finding my voice, healing from the pain, and growing to accept my perfect imperfections.

Without apologies!

It's amazing how you can be challenged to perceive life through different lenses. This entire experience equates to being in a room with beautiful flowers, unable to smell them, but afterward, you can walk throughout the room and distinctively smell each flower's unique scent. Therapy affords us the ability to approach life completely different.

To that end, therapy and my relationship with God gave me HOPE. Through this, I gained an increased trust in my intuition and my ability to love me enough not to accept anything less than what I DESERVED.

Therapy helped me to piece everything together.

I am a witness to you right now that there is power in healing! Although the process does not feel good as you are experiencing the pain and discomfort of your loss; I promise you that being aware of the stages of grief, knowing where you are in the process, finding healthy ways to express yourself, to cope, and love on yourself all leads to... *rediscovering and redefining yourself.*

"Change can be beautiful; butterflies
are the greatest proof of this."
~ Matshona Dhliwayo

THE REBIRTH:

Out of the Ashes

By Phoenixx Love, LCSW

I am an Outlier. A misguided Seeker. An Intuitive Empath.

An Enigma sent to heal others, as I continue to heal myself. There was a time I viewed myself as a bird with snow on her wings; weighted down and unable to fly. Limited by my circumstances, I did not know my voice to speak up and defend myself. I didn't know my strength or even who I was.

For so long, I was whoever people wanted me to be; to satisfy, please, appease, and use for their purposes. I was judged, ridiculed, and persecuted. People had their opinions of me; wanting to change me, pick out and consume my good parts, like selecting produce in the grocery store, and disregard what they felt was not suitable for them. No one gave a damn about how I felt. It only mattered if I could fit into their box of expectations.

Yet, buried underneath my smiles and willing heart were my pain, insecurities, and feelings of hurt and rejection. Periods of depression, anxiety, and a host of unresolved emotions would ensue and dominate my life for decades.

This chapter will not be a linear or chronological journey of my life, with all of the lessons learned along the way. It's NOT a story of another black girl becoming a statistic. Even though it could have ended that way. Instead, it is a *Fire-in-the-Hole* shot of poetic wisdom, peppered with reality, grit, and psychological absurdity that reflects the shattered mirror that once was MY Life.

ETHER

My parents were teenagers when I made my debut to the world. Dad was a heroin addict, and Mom had suffered from chronic mental health issues throughout her entire life.

I was a parentified child who had to walk on eggshells to please my mother since she was always in a perpetual state of crisis. My father was absent, only making appearances to ask for money or to antagonize my mother.

As a little black girl raised in a single parent household, I was a latchkey kid at the age of nine. I was perceptive at a young age, which helped develop my survival skills early. My mother would often call me the praying mantis because she would give me a directive, and I would pause to contemplate the request before taking action. It was a stark contrast to her impulsive approach to life, which often led us astray. My intuition and ability to stop and think often saved us.

When I was fourteen, we left our family home on Long Island due to differences within the family and moved around between Queens and Long Island.

Shabby apartments, shelters, and living with relatives.

There was very little stability; moments of normalcy, then back to chaos and confusion.

As a child, I found peace, solace, and joy in reading, music, and writing. It was an escape from the things that made me feel uncomfortable, sad, and scared. These hobbies brought comfort to the things I would ponder but could not explain or fully grasp in my young mind; experiences that had more questions than answers, yet shaped and molded my self-image and perception of the world.

For example, the time I witnessed my mother being dragged down a flight of stairs by her braids, by her then 6-foot-4 inches tall boyfriend. My mother, like me, is a small, petite woman, and her body resembled a rag doll as she cried and screamed in terror.

I desperately tried to stop him, entangled in the madness, struggling to free my mother from his grip. He was too big... too strong. I could not save her.

The same man I grew to love, who characteristically was a gentle giant. Bewildered, I could not understand when and why he turned into a raging monster, trying to kill my mother.

I WAS **helpless**...

Or, the experience of watching my brother's biological father who was like a stepdad to me, lose the cartilage of his nose in a cloth from snorting too much cocaine. My mother was frantically trying to help him, and while in his inebriated state, he fumbles around our kitchen with blood and flesh gushing from his nose. The same man who was physically abusive towards her, she was trying to save.

I WAS **confused**...

Or, maybe it was when I was fourteen years old. We had recently moved, so I decided to visit my father, only to be ignored and dismissed. He was much too preoccupied with his next "fix." As we stood in the entryway of the tenement where he resided with my stepmother and siblings, I can remember him looking out the window of the exit door, with a package of steaks in his hand. He was anxiously waiting for the dealer to arrive so that he could make his exchange. He did not hear a word I said.

I WAS **invisible...**

Or, it's THE experience that set the stage for much of my detours in life. To share this, I must go further back to when I was five years old, and a male relative took the liberty of giving me my first lesson in sex education. When I asked for help with wiping after using the bathroom, he gladly assisted. I vividly remember that this man-child violated my five-year-old body. He molested me. I was clueless. I was defenseless.

I WAS **a sex object...**

From this experience and others, I learned very early in life that boys and men want you in a subservient, vulnerable position, to objectify you, control you, and use you for their pleasure. I thought pleasuring the male species with my body was normal. After all, *what else did I have to offer?* my young mind thought. Hell, my own father did not want anything to do with me! Why would a boy or man want me in their life, other than for sex?

As a teen and young adult, I would flaunt my endowments, because after all, that was my greatest ass-et. Right?

There was no father or strong male figure to vet the men in my life. Therefore, I floundered and experimented; justifying my actions with being sexually liberated, and free to choose my lovers like I choose my outfits. I did not see any real-life examples of loving, supportive, caring father figures. I did not see many thriving marriages where both husband and wife deeply loved and respected each other.

That was not my reality.

The molestation was never discussed; as if it never happened. A part of me tucked it away deep into my subconscious, only for it to covertly resurface throughout my romantic relationships. It influenced how I viewed myself, my feelings of worth and value, as it relates to the opposite sex. I was promiscuous fairly early, and found myself in compromising situations, because of my uninhibited lifestyle.

I was seeking the love, attention, adoration, and companionship that I did not receive during my childhood.

My first love was my father. I longed for his love and attention. I felt he loved his drugs and his new family more than me. As a result, I began what seemed like a lifetime of longing, for a love that was just for me.

It's easy to feel lost or invisible when you have been taught by your parents that you are not important, or your feelings do not matter. I learned that no matter how much I achieve, what I do is not enough. I became a high achiever, or an overachiever, according to my mother. I was always striving for the best grades, participating in multiple activities, joining organizations, playing different instruments, singing in the choir—anything, and everything to get recognition from my parents—especially my father; to hear, *"I am proud of you. I love you."*

This was yearning with a dead end.

My father is a gifted artist, songwriter, and musician who plays multiple instruments. Although multi-talented, his life was unable to rise above his habits. My parents separated when I was an infant and officially divorced when I was eight. Around that time, my father attended one of my talent shows, much to my delight. I thought *I am singing a song I wrote myself. He would be so proud of me.*

He WAS there. I did see him in the audience from the stage. Did he really see me? He left abruptly before the show ended, with little recognition and without saying goodbye. I was disappointed.

As I would learn, this would not be the last time. Like I often did, I sucked it up and went on to the next achievement.

This chasing of the dream with the pursuit of acknowledgment from my father would become a recurring nightmare; ultimately an unfulfilled void I desperately spent decades trying to fill.

MASK ON

No Father. No Protector. Bad People. I am Exposed.

Who can I count on to protect me? I learned that I must guard and protect myself by any means necessary. I was a fighter. Since I was smaller than most, and the only girl living on a block full of boys, I had to be tough and defend myself. I was a tomboy that consistently had to fight battles for my younger brother and me. The tomboy evolved into an Alpha woman who never put down the proverbial gloves.

This would become a pattern in my life.

Fighting for myself, fighting for the weak and disenfranchised, always suiting up for a lifetime of battles; which God did not intend for me, and certainly did not give me the physical stature or emotional makeup for opponents to recognize.

I often shocked my opponents in both childhood fights and adult disagreements. Where I lacked physical size, He gave me ingenuity, intuition, fortitude, and a powerful spirit. No one can see these intangible qualities; therefore, I am often misunderstood or underestimated. I have been met with hostilities and sarcasm, or not taken seriously simply because I don't look the part. However, my presence is felt. My aura is colorful and alive. My spirit is soothing.

I am a natural born leader.

Still, my personality and inherent traits are incongruent with how I look. Even my voice is a dichotomy. After speaking to me on the phone, I show up, and some people are perplexed.

This is a factor I cannot change. It's how God designed me.

I often laugh and say that God had a sick sense of humor when he created me. Everything that is big about me is internal and unseen. Everything small is visible and obvious.

This disconnect regarding my appearance has also been a source of pain and rejection because people make assumptions, pass judgments, and reject what they don't understand.

Acceptance is based on what is deemed normal, standard or status quo. I guess I am supposed to be timid, shy and powerless. But I'm not. A sense of belonging has often eluded me because I don't necessarily fit anywhere; I don't categorize well. Developing a healthy love and appreciation for all of me required years of work. I had a warped view of love.

Even for myself.

Unconditional love did not exist in my world. There were always conditions. The only person I knew who loved me unconditionally and I could feel it deep in my soul was my paternal grandmother. She was the mother figure in my life, and her love was pure. She accepted and loved me for who I was, and I loved her dearly. I spent most of my childhood under my grandmother's roof. I enjoyed being her helper with household chores—cooking, cleaning, and hanging clothes to dry in the sun.

My job was to pass the clothespins as I listened to her sing and hum. We would walk to the neighborhood fruit stand singing songs, telling knock-knock jokes, and laughing. I loved helping her to stir cake mix, knead dough and shuck peas. *Yes,* she was that grandma. I now understand that that was my first experience of mindfulness activities that I would later use to help countless children.

At night, we would curl up on her bed and watch monster movies or comedy shows, like *The Honeymooners* or *Sanford and Son.* When I was with her, I knew everything would be okay. She was my number one supporter and cheerleader; filling the gap my parents were incapable of fulfilling.

When I was a junior in college, my beloved grandmother died of cancer. This was a pivotal time in my development and maturity. I was nineteen years old and embarking on adulthood. School was always a place where I had a sense of control and mastery; however, her death made me feel like I had no control over anything.

When I got the call at school that my grandmother's health was declining, I took the first train back home to be with her. Much to my dismay, by the time I arrived, she was gone.

I did not get the chance to say goodbye.

Sitting in our family's cramped apartment, in the kitchen/sleep area/living room, I remember feeling numb with disbelief. Her death changed me. I went through an extended period where I was a rebel without a cause, reckless and foolish at times. I didn't care. I found comfort in my madness, numbing my pain and shame with drinking, sex, and partying.

It had become an extended time of distraction from dealing with my heartbreak; while avoiding my shame and attenuation. When my grandmother left this earth, a piece of me died, and there was a shift in my spirit.

 My mask was on.

BURIED TREASURE

Over the years, I participated in therapy with a psychotherapist with little progress. We only scratched the surface, never addressing the core issues that had a stronghold over my life. I attended church regularly but was merely sitting in the pews sinking every Sunday. I was ritualistically performing all of the formalities with NO power, NO results.

Tuesday prayer and Wednesday Bible study did not help either, and what I learned is that religious ritual was not the answer for me. My relationship with God went through periods of depth and some power only to dwindle whenever a crisis would hit my household. I had my trials of backsliding. Although I knew the Bible, the guiding principles of Christianity, and how to pray in times of trouble, something was still missing. Something that would speak to my inner woman, get to my core and dig out what was holding me hostage; breaking the chains.

Freedom.

It was not until I was at a breaking point in my life that real change occurred. I was sitting in my bedroom, staring out the window, reflecting on a haunting past and dismal present, and contemplating my reason for being here. I was at an all-time low. It was Mother's Day.

Since I often felt like an orphan on this earth, it was one of my least favorite holidays. I always thought of my grandmother on this day, more than others. I was broken and grappling with my existence. I was depressed and questioning my worth and value. Adults often make a mess out of a child's life and leave it for them to unravel and clean up in their adulthood. I felt life was unfair.

I can remember lying prostrate on the floor, sobbing uncontrollably, asking for God to just acknowledge me, my pain, and my shame. Rescue me and help me not to feel this way anymore. Deliver me from this spirit of heaviness. Give me a reason to live and see another day. Help me make sense out of everything I had been through.

What is my purpose? What am I supposed to be doing?

I cried out, *"WHY AM I HERE?!"*

At that moment, I felt the warmth of light over me; a comforting peace surrounded me, and my spirit felt lifted up. The only way I can explain it is God dried my tears. I felt His presence, and He told me, *"You would never be depressed again. You would help heal those who are downtrodden, broken and living in despair."* He said that He would use my hurt, pain, and shame to help others who are struggling in their lives. I had a mission, a calling that is important and that only I can do. It was time for me to unveil my past and heal, so I can heal and bless others.

I was reminded that I could not pour from an empty cup, which is what I had been doing that led to my breakdown. You cannot *pour new wine into old wineskins*. It was time to release all that had been weighing me down. It's like withdrawing from an account that is already in the red. It was time to make deposits and get back into the black. The alarm was ringing. I knew I needed to seek above and beyond professional help.

Above and beyond religion.

I required more. I required Healing AND Deliverance.

With relentless intent, a few months later I signed up for Iyanla Vanzant's *Wonder Woman Weekend*. A program I had known about for many years, always wanted to go to but would talk myself out of it for a variety of reasons.

Not this time. I had a Divine appointment.

I remember jumping in my car on a cool fall morning and making that drive south on the 95 to Maryland. I was determined to get my healing. I didn't know what to expect, because the program was designed with no itinerary and very little information. This was intentional for participants to come with an open mind. It was a life-changing experience for me that would begin my healing process and give me a deeper look at spiritual and holistic interventions.

The experiential exercises that were used during the weekend were groundbreaking. They helped me, and the other attendees dig deep, pull out the suppressed emotions, and open up Pandora's Box. In other words, it was time to finally submit to the Divine and confront the ugly part of my life that I had been suppressing for so long; which had been holding me in bondage for decades, keeping me stuck and unable to realize my dreams.

I was ready to release all of the baggage I had been carrying around in my mind, body, and spirit as a heavy burden. It was time to let it go... time to surrender.

And, I did.

One of the healing exercises was releasing our Shadow Self and unveiling our True Self. We were given a name tag upon arrival that we chose out of a box and wore throughout the weekend. My Shadow name was FORGOTTEN. This label strongly resonated with me; considering the road I had traveled.

At the end of the weekend, there is a renaming ceremony, where we discard the Shadow name and retrieve our new True name. My True Self's name was DEVOTION. I cried with joy because this transition spoke to my soul and described who I aspired to be. Like many, I was suffering from Identity theft. Unchecked and Unhealed trauma robs your Soul. I was taking back what was rightfully mine.

This moment was surreal.

Iyanla was enthralled with this new name for me; giving me the biggest Auntie hug and kiss on the cheek, and what felt like the longest stare, as if she could see within me.

Affirmation.

I felt like I had won the lottery. It was a tender moment because I felt like I was born again. When I left the divine space, my wings were lighter.

This was an eye-opening turning point in my life. I had unpacked over thirty years of baggage in one weekend. Although I was a little open and raw, I felt empowered. I felt strong.

And, I began to draw lines in the sand with overbearing and draining relationships; removing people from my life, setting boundaries with whom I couldn't sever ties, and resigning from a toxic job.

My life was going in the right direction.

As a trained therapist, I was clear this was the beginning of my journey. This would be a lifetime of restorative work and repair to provide a protective balm of healing over my raw and exposed wiring. So, I went on a quest.

"What you seek is seeking you."
~Rumi

I was on a quest to discover who I truly was. To reclaim what was lost. Seeking answers for all of the questions that crowd my mind daily. I wanted to silence the noise in my head: the ancient secrets, the suppressed memories, and the ghosts of the past. I needed to deal with my demons once and for all.

However, you cannot kill demons and vampires unless you shine the light on them.

It was time to draw back the curtains.

First, this expedition led me to two gifted energy healers and yoga instructors, who later became my mentors and spiritual guides. I learned more about the effects of trauma and stress on my mind and body, focusing on the energy centers/meridians; also known as Chakras. I was taught how the brain and the central nervous system play a vital role to the restoration of every part of our body, cells, and organs, especially as it relates to achieving balance, alignment, and overall wellness goals.

I incorporated more intentional movement and eastern healing techniques such as Yoga, Tai Chi, Meditation, Breath-work, and Acupuncture in my routine health regimen. I started altering my eating habits, removing certain foods that spiked my blood sugar levels. I had been diagnosed a year before with being pre-diabetic and was prescribed Metformin.

It made me feel awful. I knew I had to make some physical changes in both movement and diet. Which I did; however, there was still an identity and spiritual void that was left unfulfilled.

At the time, I was attending a church that I loved, but I still felt a spiritual disconnect. Like a fish out of water. My prayer life was not as strong as it should have been. Consequently, there were prayers, but not enough manifestations and depth in my spiritual connection to God and people.

Most of my relationships were superficial and esoteric at best, including my relationship with myself, and to some degree, my Divine Creator. It was important to me that this area of my life not be left unfinished and vulnerable. I feared that old thoughts and behaviors would return if I did not strengthen my spiritual life. I could not take that risk, and I refused to go backward.

I had come too far.

THE AWAKENING

My spiritual journey and goals to improve my health led me to *Queen Afua Sacred Woman* program out of Brooklyn, N.Y. *Sacred Woman* is a 12-week Rites of passage program that teaches women from the African Diaspora how to heal themselves—mind, body, soul, and spirit—using Holistic health practices and natural medicine.

It culminates with an awe-inspiring Ascension that celebrates the graduates and educates family, friends, and community about Kemetic Spirituality principles via 12 Gateways that is the heart and soul of the program.

The program promotes a healthy plant-based lifestyle, prosperous relationships, prayer, meditation, and maintaining a balanced, harmonious environment.

The goal is to develop women as practitioners and healers to further the cause of Health and wellness, entrepreneurship, sense of community, cooperative economics, love, and positivity. We can heal and empower ourselves, family, community and ultimately the world.

After the 12-week intensive, by the time I walked across the stage for Ascension, I had given birth to Phoenixx Love. Phoenixx was NOT the girl who struggled for years with her identity, worth, value, pain, and shame. She was now open to new possibilities and ready to continue her healing; while helping others to heal.

Phoenixx is a beautiful black Queen on Fire for Healing, Love, Truth, and Justice. I had survived and made it through the peaks and valleys of life. Rebirth. I am no longer a bird with snow on my wings, but a powerful Phoenix ready to soar and help distressed souls. I am a Sacred Woman.

I am a Healer.

This was a pivotal time. As I said *"yes"* to me, the doors began to open. I launched my Holistic Healing practice *Healer's Haven* to help individuals struggling with emotional turmoil, trauma, relationships, and spiritual warfare. I completed my first book *"If*

I Should Die Before I Wake: Your Journey to Awakening Your Calling" and published it as a healing tool to share with the world. I realized it took me ten years before I could sit down and write my first book. I had so many blockages and was closed off to receiving God's downloads.

Finally, my mind is liberated. TUA NTR

I recognized and often share with my clients, this is exactly what happens when you are disconnected and out of alignment. You cannot move forward without dying to your former, broken self and being born again to your revitalized and healed true self. This is a process; often a painful, ugly process... but, necessary.

It is both spiritual and holistic health—mind, body, soul, and spirit. I knew my calling was to use my training and skills in the mental health field while incorporating vital spiritual guidance and holistic health practices. Help for individuals who are lost, broken, and suffering from past trauma, emotional turmoil, and generational curses.

For over a year, I immersed myself into gaining a deeper understanding of how the body and mind works. I made me a priority and invested in a variety of advanced training and certification courses in energy healing, new generation evidence-based practices, neuroscience studies, reflexology, and various types of yoga and meditation classes.

As I gained new knowledge to expand my practice, I prayed to God to send me spiritual guides and mentors that will not only help me along my personal journey but also provide guidance and wisdom to me as a Holistic Health Practitioner.

He answered me, sending me not one, but four mentors with different levels of expertise for each aspect of my development.

I was rich in wisdom, knowledge, and awareness; finally able to connect all of the dots to see the bigger picture that the Divine had illustrated just for my life. My eyes were opening to a new reality that I didn't know existed. When I reflect, it took twenty years of falling down and getting back up, and a string of unfortunate events, before I finally discovered ME… the real, Authentic me.

Not who everyone thought I should be, but who God created me to be. The reality is that she was always there, buried under a mountain of emotional rubble. My eyes always saw something different. My mind always perceived something in a unique way. My view of the world was tainted, a little twisted, sometimes dark, mysterious with hints of light and beauty. I always felt like an alien from out of space, peculiar, oddly unique, and set apart, until I finally accepted that I was DIFFERENT, and it's OKAY!

A misfit with a purpose. Strange Fruit.

But God led me to *The Sacred Woman* program, where I am surrounded by a tribe of misfits with a purpose. Some people say Unicorns. I say Shining Beings. God's special creatures plucked out of miry pits and shined up, like a diamond from coal, for Divine work on this earth.

MASK OFF

"I was lost, but now I am found. I was blind, but now I see. Thank you for saving a wretch like me." I am grateful for the journey that I have been on. I am grateful for all of the trials and tribulations that have shaped me into the woman I am today; the ability to heal others through my intuitive wisdom and gifts that were hand-picked for me—a Divine Masterpiece.

God called and anointed me to touch people and transform lives; to lift my voice and sing MY song. Recite my poem. Write my Story. And, Reveal my inner strength.

From the time I was in college, I set out on a mission to serve. It started with organizing a tutoring and mentoring program with the local intermediate school near my undergraduate college; creating awareness on my campus about Social Justices, volunteering with Domestic Violence victims and the homeless.

It progressed to Community leadership positions and Youth mentorship in my hometown; paying it forward, all before earning a living as a trained and licensed mental health clinician.

Right after college, I took a detour and landed in corporate America for ten years. Here is where I fell in love with Human behavior, traveling across the States conducting consumer and market research. However, because I was destined to work in the mental health and human services field, the road led me back to this field, at the right time, for the right season. Destiny ultimately summoned and ushered me into the very place I am today. It was a path that required my valleys in life, as well as my mountains.

I now understand that.

Early in my mental health career, I was led to work with children and adolescents with backgrounds similar to mine: trauma, sexual abuse, and domestic violence that branded their young minds and spirits with self-loathing, low esteem, and internalized wounds that required extensive therapy, love, and support to heal.

I know this all too well. As a therapist, it is important to me to provide a safe haven; understanding and applying the intricacies of human behavior not only from a psychological perspective but a holistic perspective. I have studied theorist Erik Erikson's Eight Stages of Psychosocial Development as a guide to human functioning, according to chronological growth and development. My analytical mind closely associates my own experiences and my clients' with Andrew Maslow and use of his *Hierarchy of Needs*.

This theoretical model helps connect the dots between our childhood experiences and how we function as adults. When those basic needs of safety, security, and sustenance are not met in childhood, a pathological pattern in adulthood that can be a barrier to optimal living will be prevalent.

According to Maslow, one cannot fully self-actualize without the strong foundation at the base of his model: "sense of security" and "sense of belonging." These two areas were unhealed and repeatedly showed up in my life as unmet needs. My life story is a prime example of the longitudinal research study, Adverse Childhood Experiences (ACES). The research indicates that if you have an ACES score of four or more traumatic events, you are at high risk of physical and mental health conditions that can lead to higher mortality rates.

My score was eight. I was heading down this road of self-destruction that forced me to make a choice, not only for me but also for my family. A choice to heal on my terms and to restore equanimity through a combination of therapy, spiritual practices, and holistic interventions. This path was necessary for God to use me on this earth as a Soul Healer and Kingdom builder.

My capricious walk in life has prepared me to be the living example for countless souls that will come and tell their story; stories of trauma, victimization, the perpetrators, the broken system, and the injustices that prevail every day. I leverage my voids, my sexual abuse, and being a witness of violence, to fuel a deep passion for helping young women and girls who are victims of familial abuse, child sex trafficking, and domestic violence; including teen dating abuse. I have also learned over time that there is an increasing number of boys and men who share these experiences in record numbers. However, it is hidden and kept secret for obvious reasons.

I believe part of my mission is to shine a light on the Truth through awareness of these infractions and serious offenses, especially in black communities, so victims can get the help they need and move from victim to victor.

When you have walked through hell, come out the other side with a little soot and smoke, but still standing, you must commend yourself and celebrate that you are still here.

Why? *Because God has a greater plan for your life.*

Don't allow the negative experiences from your past to dictate your future. Use those experiences as fuel for your fire. Your power lies in your ability to survive the experience and still come out shining. One thing I have gleaned from my journey is that all of the experiences; good, bad, and indifferent, can be used to bless others. It is a choice that one has to be willing to make. It is a step forward that one has to be willing to take. It is in remembering your resiliency that you will find the courage to stand in the face of adversity, time and time again.

Recovery is this: I peeled back the layers of the smelly onion called my life and evolved into a fragrant Lotus Blossom.

I exposed the hidden parts, the faulty wiring, and challenged my vulnerabilities and sensibilities to heal myself using Holistic

Health practices, so that God could use me according to the blue-print He designed.

Holistic Healing is an excavation and exploration of self: mentally, emotionally, physically and spiritually.

At **Healer's Haven,** my work with clients involves ripping off the band-aid, allowing the scars and wounds to breathe, grow a scab, and reveal a new surface. It's a process; not a quick fix. It's not a prescriptive one-shot transaction like when you go to the doctor for an ailment.

I work with clients by meeting them where they are; forming a therapeutic alliance over time that yields long-lasting results, not anecdotal temporary solutions. It is a step-by-step customized transformative process that explores a healthy balance of psycho-analysis, narrative therapy, and holistic therapeutic interventions especially, to address traumatic cases.

Out of the ashes, I was a tortured soul with many battle wounds and scars that are now healing. I was stuck in neutral; going no-where. I had to expose what was hidden in the dark and allow the healing oil to do what was necessary to restore those wounded areas and stabilize my life. Although I have experienced loss on so many levels, by the grace of God, I have found the strength to rebuild and put the pieces back together.

I had to remember who I was, reach back to my early days of innocence, and heal my inner child, as I do with many of my clients. The unhealed child will always show up as the dysfunc-tional, broken adult. In these precarious days, I am called and anointed for this time to provide therapeutic healing solutions. I am equipped and destined to help each willing soul build the bridge from a fragmented past to a redeemed present, to a reclaimed future, for generations to come.

In the same way, it is important to examine your story, find the themes, and start to dissect those negative schemas; then you can tell your story from the vantage point of the healed version of you. He has called many of you to do something trailblazing in this season.

Are You Ready?

Let's start a wellness revolution together...
Healing One Soul at a Time

Ase'

SAVING MY YOUNGER SELF

By Nicole Thompson, Ed. S.

"And I think that vulnerability is the cornerstone of confidence. Because you have to allow yourself to take risk, to be open, to live as a wholehearted person."

-Oprah Winfrey

For many years, I was angry with and resentful of my mom. I couldn't understand how a mother of five children could take her life and leave them to fend for themselves. Furthermore, drink during her entire pregnancy, which caused my youngest sister to be premature. I believed with all my heart that she was selfish and could not possibly love my siblings and me because she left us.

It was not until my early 20s that I realized it was not selfishness. Somehow, a couple of my friends and I had gotten on the topic of moms, and I lashed out in anger, as I usually would, concerning mine.

At that moment, my best friend told me I shouldn't be angry with my mom because she was depressed. That was the first time I ever heard someone use that term when referring to my mom.

This had never crossed my mind, simply because I had never taken the time to process the real reason why she left me. It was truly an epiphany for me at that moment, and I very slowly began to release my anger and, to some extent, attempt to understand her mental health issues and the effects of trauma.

As a child, my siblings and I witnessed some of the worst moments of my mom's life. We witnessed her abusive marriage with my dad for years in which he was emotionally and physically abusive to her. At the time, our lives mirrored the 1984 movie *The Burning Bed,* in which the wife kills her husband by setting the bed on fire while he is sleeping after he severely abuses her on many occasions.

Watching the movie with my mom was like watching our life on the big screen. The slaps, punches, hair pulling, and verbal abuse were all too familiar. My mom finally found the courage to leave not too long after my brother threatened to kill my dad if he hit her again.

After leaving my dad, we moved into my grandma's two-bedroom house in North Philly. This area of the city was impoverished and had all the underpinnings of poverty, such as drugs, violence, and a general sense of hopelessness. It didn't take long for my mom to succumb to such an environment.

Shortly after we settled in, my mom and grandma began to argue quite often, so my grandma went to stay with her sister. The fact that their relationship was already strained may have contributed to the arguments.

My grandma had my mom when she was a teenager, so my great grandma was more of the caregiver than my grandma.

I realized my mom never forgave *her* mom, as evidenced by her lack of respect. For example, she always called her by her first name. At the time, I didn't realize anything was wrong with calling your mom by her first name. In my young mind, I thought this was how adults referred to their parents.

Of course, now I know such not to be true and realize that there was trauma in my mom's life dating back to being born to a teenage mom.

Time went on, and my mom started a relationship with a new guy from the neighborhood. That relationship seemed to take precedence in her life, and her children seemed to be an afterthought. She would leave us in the house, sometimes late at night, to be with him. I never knew where they were; I just knew that my mom wasn't where she needed to be—home with her children.

To make matters worse, there were times when he beat me for acting up. One time, he beat me with an extension cord while holding me upside down by my ankles. This left me wondering why my mom would allow this to happen when this man wasn't even my stepdad. He attempted to beat one of my brothers as well, but my brother wasn't having it.

One dreadful night, my mom got a visitor informing her that her boyfriend had been killed. He had gotten into a heated argument with his dad like many times before, but this time his dad stabbed him in the heart, and he died.

To make matters worse, my brother was a witness to the atrocious event. Although the courts wanted him to testify, my mom and grandma refused to let him do so because he was barely a teenager at the time. Now, my mom was left to bear such news and carry their unborn child without any hopes of the baby ever knowing its father.

As one can imagine, she did not take the news well. Shortly after, she slipped into a very deep depression. She stopped eating, and all she would do was drink.

My siblings and I became her gophers for buying her liquor from the speakeasy across the street from us. We had also become our own keepers because she neglected us. She even neglected our baby sister-to-be by "nourishing" her with nothing but alcohol. These habits led my mom to premature birth, and my sister was born months early, weighing a little over a pound.

The neglect my siblings and I suffered seemed insurmountable. Our house was always filthy and had so many roaches that it would make any normal person gag. There was never a time that I didn't have to battle with the roaches to eat because they were in the refrigerator and cabinets. I would always cringe when I saw them crawling in and out of the boxes or across the food.

We had very little food to begin with, so it was either eat what was there or starve. After all, my mom wasn't going shopping, so we made do with what we had.

It was during this time that I saw "albino roaches."

The first time I saw one, I thought it had come from the flour bag, but as I checked around, we didn't have flour. Although five of us lived there at the time, it seemed like we were outnumbered by the roaches by fifty to one. It was as if they ruled the place and we were just visitors. There were occasions when I went to school and one of them would crawl out my backpack or book. I would quickly glance around the room to see if anyone saw it before I smashed it.

To be honest, the roaches were probably the least of our worries. My brothers and I used to spend the night over at the neighbor's house quite often because we were friends with her children. One time, my friend and I were headed downstairs for something when we saw her mom and friends smoking crack. We snooped down quietly and watched in shock until her mom caught us and yelled at us to go back upstairs.

Terrified by what we saw and that we were caught, we hurried off back into the bedroom and closed the door.

Another time, we were all in the living room, and their mom was arguing with her son. She was standing over him while he sat on the couch. All of a sudden, she called him a pussy and smacked him on the side of the head with her pistol. Blood trickled from the side of his head, and he started to cry.

My heart ached for him as I sat and watched, paralyzed, at a loss for words. The sad part about this all is that I believed it was normal because this was the life I lived every day.

Approximately three months after my little sister's birth, I woke up in the middle of the night because she was crying very loudly. Since we only had two bedrooms, my siblings and I rotated who slept in my mom's room.

That night, it was my turn. My baby sister always slept with her since she was so young. When I awoke, I saw my mom lying on my sister, which apparently was the reason for her cry. I nudged my mom and told her that she was lying on my sister. She didn't move. I shook her a little harder and called her name a little louder.

No answer.

At this point, panic started to move through my body, and I felt myself begin to tremble and become terrified. So many thoughts were racing through my head. I flashed back to earlier that night before we went to bed; my mom sat all her kids around her and told us she was going to die that night. I cried and pleaded with her not to say such things, but she did not change her story.

This couldn't be true! Mommy, NO!

I also remembered that my mom's friend had come over a day or so before to show me how to check a pulse. I was upstairs, and my mom called me in the living room to learn the lesson. I was very inquisitive as a child, and at the time I wanted to be a doctor, so I thought it was the coolest thing ever.

As the neighbor was teaching me the proper way to do it, she had me practice on my mom's wrist. She told me to use my index and middle finger and demonstrated exactly on the wrist where her pulse would be found. She also told me to never use my thumb because it has its own pulse and to check on the neck directly under the chin if I couldn't find a pulse on the wrist.

Since I was such a great student, I found it on the first try. My mom and her friend commended me, and I walked away feeling proud and accomplished. As I was going through all this in my mind, I wished, once again, that I was taking my mom's pulse for practice. Unfortunately, I wasn't.

In the bed, I rolled her all the way over on her back and held her wrist in my hand. My heart felt like it was beating out of my chest and my head was starting to pound. I placed my pointer and middle finger on her wrist and felt for her pulse, just as I did during the lesson.

I felt nothing.

Holding back tears, I placed my fingers on her neck.

Still... nothing.

Full of pain and fear, I jumped off the bed, ran into the next room, woke my brothers, and that's when it happened. Tears streamed down my young eyes, and I spoke the unfathomable, *"I think Mommy is dead."*

What happened immediately after that is a blur. The next thing I remember was my neighbor coming up the street, telling us to clean up all the liquor bottles laying around the rooms because the ambulance was on the way.

Again, what followed those instructions is a total blur.

The day after my mom passed, I stared in the mirror and thought that I was dreaming. For sure, I had to be dreaming. After all, there was no way my mom actually died last night in between my little sister and me. I pinched myself and felt it. Maybe that was just a coincidence. I slapped myself and felt that, too. Suddenly, a crushing feeling went through my heart, and I felt like the life was being sucked out of me. I felt that familiar feeling all over again - panic.

My heart once more started racing, I felt heat move through my young body, and I started to cry. That feeling sat there with me and weighed on me like a ton of rocks. My new reality was that I was a motherless child at the age of eight.

Death wasn't new to me because our family had experienced it not too long before when my mom's boyfriend was murdered. However, this wasn't someone I just met; this was my mom, the source of my existence.

So many thoughts and questions went through my head. However, I was too afraid to ask any of them because I knew my grandma was in excruciating pain, and I didn't want to make it worse by asking a million questions. *Is my grandma going to raise us now? Will we ever see our dad again? When am I going back to school? What will everyone say when they find out?*

Nighttime fell upon us, and it was time for us to go to bed. For some reason, and, unfortunately, I will never know the answer to why my grandma told me to go to sleep in the same room and bed where I had just awakened to find my mother's lifeless body. When she instructed me to do so, I began to yell and cry uncontrollably, saying, *"I don't ever wanna go in that room again!"*

At this point, I believe she realized how insensitive and cruel it was to request such because she told me to sleep in the other room. I lay in between my brothers, still shaken and terrified about what we all as siblings experienced the night before. None of us talked about anything; we just lay there until we all fell asleep.

Days later, my mom's funeral occurred. My grandma got us all dressed up and headed to the church, which was around the corner. The immediate family sat on the front row just a couple of feet in front of her casket. Since she was an only child, it only included my grandma and us (her children).

I know that this was done out of respect, but it was more painful for me to continuously watch my dead mom lie in that casket an entire funeral service. As I sat, I looked around for my dad, but there was no sight of him. I hadn't seen him since we had moved in with my grandma, which was at least two years prior. The service continued with kind words about my mom and mentions of her five children and the mother she was leaving behind.

She was only 33 years old.

At times, I would stop crying just long enough to catch my breath, but then I would be caught with another heart-wrenching moment. The pastor's daughter sang with so much feeling and intensity that I could not help but cry uncontrollably. She sang the exact way I would have if I could sing. It was as if she felt my pain and was able to relay it for me.

The time came when everyone lined up to view the body. When I looked at her, she didn't look the same. She had on makeup. She never wore makeup. With tears rolling down my eyes, I continued to stare, thinking that this could not be my mom. I guess I was standing there too long, since my grandma told me to kiss her and return to my seat so that others could pay their respects.

I kissed her cheek, and to my surprise, it felt like kissing a cold concrete wall. Kissing my mom made me feel worse because, in that instant, I realized that the body lying in the coffin was no longer my mommy, just a lifeless shell. Her soul and her being had passed on.

About a week later, my siblings and I went to live with my dad. Just like that, we were swept up like a whirlwind, our lives turned upside down, but business continued as normal.

Our transition to our dad's house was seamless in that nothing we had been through was discussed. We simply made the move and life went on as if none of the horrific events leading up to us moving with our dad had ever happened. Nonetheless, I was so happy to see my dad again because it had seemed like an eternity. I wondered if my brother felt the same way since the last real contact we had with him was when he threatened my dad's life.

My grandma kept my baby sister since she was not his. It was weird to live apart from my newborn sister; our bond was just forming, and then we were separated without much notice. Although we lived with my dad, we would visit our grandma and baby sister every other weekend.

My grandma would briefly mention my mom occasionally, but we never had an open conversation about what had transpired. I guess it was too painful for my grandma to be vulnerable about losing her one and only child. Seeing her five grandchildren lose their mom.

One thing I will never forget my grandma mentioning is that my mom called my grandma's pastor before she passed and was "saved." Was my grandma only telling me this to save face? Did my grandma know what took me almost thirty years to figure out? My mom committed suicide.

Of course, this is something that has never been discussed or "proven," but reflecting on the events lead me to believe that she did indeed take her own life.

I transferred to my new elementary school, where no one knew me. I didn't have trouble making friends and seemed to find a few quite easily. The only problem was since they were just getting to know me they assumed I had a mom.

What they thought were innocent conversations, were like bandages being repeatedly ripped off a gaping wound. I was so ashamed that I no longer had a mom that I would lie. Pretending that my mom was still alive became the norm, and it wasn't until high school that I finally opened up and told my friends that my mom had passed.

"For the wise know the truth;
in helping others we help ourselves..."
-Napoleon Hill

The events leading up to my mom's death were most certainly capable of pushing anyone into depression. Although I understood such, I still had a long recovery process that took many years. One day, not too long ago, I looked at my mom's obituary. For the first time, I looked at her picture with admiration. There was finally no trace of resentment or anger.

I have lived, and have struggled and overcome, but not nearly as much as she did. When I think back to the trauma she experienced in her short lifetime, I commend her for her strength and wish she could have lived to tell her own story. Since she didn't, I feel compelled to share her story—my story—in hopes of helping others with comparable pasts.

Growing up in a traumatic, neglectful environment led me to become a school psychologist because I so desperately wanted to help children who experienced similar situations. I remembered all the pain and neglect I went through as a child, and wanted, somehow, to alleviate other children's pain. Although I know total alleviation isn't possible, I could at least be there to help them through the trauma and get them to the point of healing much sooner than the 30+ years that it took me to do so partly on my own. The reason I say "partly" on my own is that I didn't start the healing process until I began my work in helping others to heal.

There I was, years later, and my life had come full circle. I was now working in the same school district that served me as a child.

Walking the halls, looking around, seeing all those faces, reminded me of my childhood.

It also led me to remember some of the trauma my childhood friends and I had gone through. I kept telling myself, "I am these children. I have to do right by them."

At the time, I didn't know exactly what that would be, but I knew I stepped into the role to get one step closer. After all, I know for sure that all children need a caring adult, a champion to be there with them through hard times. After my mom passed, I vividly remember my third-grade teacher giving me two jumbo coloring books and a box of sixty-four crayons.

Although that may seem like a small gesture to many, it meant the world to me, and I will never forget it. That is the type of adult I want to be; one who cares enough to have an impact on a child's life, even if I don't realize it.

I am almost certain that at the time, my teacher had no clue she would impact my life forever and be one of the driving forces behind my career.

As the years passed in my role as a school psychologist, I began to establish a good rapport with some of the students. They would come to my office, often to talk light-heartedly, and to be vulnerable about different matters they were experiencing at home. I felt honored that the students trusted me enough to share some of their deepest secrets and pain, without ever being coaxed into sharing.

It was during these moments that I was constantly reminded of the trauma that occurs in so many of our children's lives. I also realized that like myself, many of these children kept their pain to themselves, built a wall through some type of coping mechanism, and were never encouraged to seek help. Sadly, many of their coping mechanisms involved extreme externalizing behaviors which often result in serving time in the prison system, and ultimately being labeled as Emotionally Disturbed (ED), such as selling drugs. ED is an umbrella term used within the school system to describe students who don't fit the cultural norms of a socially/emotionally healthy student.

My question is, how can they fit within the norms if their lives are totally outside of what is normal? Their home lives certainly aren't, and many of the environments in which they live aren't either. I will be the first to attest that living in poverty is a constant struggle of its own.

The more I witnessed one student after the next come to my office, living through a personal hell at home, I began to think about the question I had posed because it deeply bothered me. The empathy that I felt for these teens is what inspired me to start an all-female empowerment group. The reason behind mentoring females, in particular, is that I believe that in order to make a gen-erational change, it has to begin with the creators of life.

Of course, I also enjoyed working with male teens and did my best to inspire them as well, but my passion is with females. My passion is to save my younger self; just thinking of my own family, riddled with generational trauma dating back to my grandma having my mom when she was still a teenager. And, though I don't know the story behind it, I can safely assume that this is what caused many of my mom's adult issues.

I never knew my grandpa and never heard my mom mention him, which leads me to believe that my mom had some daddy issues she was dealing with. This further explains why she stayed with my dad for so long in an abusive, unhealthy marriage.

She didn't have someone outside of her immediate environment to nurture her, teach her a new way of life, and encourage her to dream big and go for those dreams. My mom and grandma didn't have a great woman who knew better and pushed them to do better. They didn't have a therapist or a mentor to help guide them to greatness. In my personal opinion, you need both to get you to live your best life.

What I know for sure is that I am thankful for the life that was given to me. Many might not understand my reasoning for such a statement, but, without those adverse childhood experiences, I would not be in pursuit of my dreams to help develop emotionally healthy, educated generations of females. It is now my purpose to break typical matriarchal roles at such an early age and develop strong, confident, female leaders who know themselves before they get to know what gender roles they should identify with.

My journey requires that I keep an open heart, to keep growing, and to keep pushing beyond uncomfortable feelings, while encouraging our girls to do so as well.

As I grow, my girls grow... and, we grow together.

DON'T GET IT TWISTED!

By Nydia E. Guity, LCSW

Who am I?

I've always felt like that was a cliché question, and my answer has traditionally been to say what I think people want to hear; saying just enough so I can go back to being introverted and minding my business.

I am the oldest of five children, born and raised in Bronx, New York. My parents are from Guadalupe (Funda), Honduras and I identify as Garifuna. Garifunas are descendants of African, Arawak and Black Caribs. The Garifuna people are mostly on the coast of Central American countries, which include Honduras, Guatemala, Belize, and Nicaragua.

Phenotypically, I am a black woman. Linguistically, I speak two and a half languages, with Spanish being my first language.

Despite being born in the United States, I didn't speak English until I learned it in the fifth grade. My parents spoke enough English to get by. Garifuna I've understood my whole life, but I am not fluent yet. When I was younger, being black and speaking Spanish made me feel like an alien. The African American kids in school called me 'Spanish,' and the Latino kids expressed that I wasn't Latina enough because of my brown skin.

As a child and into my adolescence, explaining to my peers that I was Garifuna felt like a history lesson I didn't want to teach repeatedly. Speaking Garifuna as a child wasn't a priority, so I settled and responded in Spanish when my parents spoke to me in Garifuna and left it at that. I can think back to so many instances in my life, where I was either mistaken for another ethnic group or assumed that I didn't understand the language being used at any given moment.

On paper, I am a licensed clinical social worker (LCSW). I have a Bachelor's Degree in Social Work from the University of Vermont (UVM) and a Master's Degree in Clinical Social Work from Fordham University, graduating one month before my twenty-third birthday. Sharing my academic accomplishments has always been a source of joy; it's an easy part of myself to share.

When things go well, you talk about it with confidence, PRIDE, and bass in your voice. But, what you don't know about me is that even with this fancy Master's Degree and years of experience working as a therapist servicing people who have struggled with domestic violence and all kinds of trauma, I would not be immune to the emotional, physical, and sexual mistreatment that I was to experience once I moved to Atlanta, Georgia in September 2015.

Let's take a step back.

What happened?!

Relax and gather up your favorite snacks because, in this chapter, I am going to share with you my journey to regaining the health of my hair from within.

A woman's glory is in her hair. It has volume, length and flows in the wind. When I get my hair done, my confidence reaches the heavens and how I show up in the world is a little different. When I leave the hair salon, I feel like I radiate goddess vibes of elegance, grace, and strength.

The man in my life at the time absorbed my goddess vibes and loved every bit of my natural hair! We met in September 2011 online and then face to face in October of that year.

We dated on and off and then reconnected in November 2014. We reminisced about the good times we shared before and new memories that we could create. I am from the Bronx, New York and was living there at the time that we were dating. He was in the military and stationed in Alexandria, Virginia. We scheduled our visits once a month, and during one of my trips to visit him, we planned a trip to Atlanta to shop around for a home.

Although I am not a morning person, on that Saturday morning, I remember waking early. It was Valentine's Day, and his warm, soft kisses on my forehead were a pleasant good morning just before getting myself ready for our long drive from Alexandria, Virginia to Atlanta. He drove the whole way, and I noticed that he was very affectionate; more than usual.

For most of the ride, his hand held mine.

We stopped at a gas station to stretch, and as I was waiting for him to pay for our snacks, he hugged me tightly. At that point, I stopped trying to figure out what was up and let myself enjoy all of the chocolate lovin' I was getting!

Not much later, we arrived in Hampton, Georgia. As we were unloading our stuff from his car, I discovered a silver box in my coat pocket. I looked at it and thought *what's this and who put it here?*

I opened the box, and inside was a smaller black velvet box. So, I opened the black box and there it was... a stunning diamond ring!

Turning in disbelief, I saw him standing right behind me, smiling. He said, "It was supposed to be a surprise. I wanted you to find it while we were driving so I could ask you."

Laughing, my response was, "That's not asking."

Still smiling, but saying nothing, he walked away from me, and we ended up going to view a few homes as if nothing had happened. Later that night, as we were talking about moving in together, he brought up the ring. I just kept saying that I wouldn't answer until I was formally asked.

Later that evening, at exactly 10:18 p.m., while we were sitting on the couch, he faced me and asked me to be his wife.

I said, "Yes!"

It was that 'girly yes' when your neck is tilted sideways, followed by a really big smile that makes your cheeks hurt. The engagement was special to me; it was just us. No cameras, pictures, or props displaying to the world what love should look like. When that three-carat princess-cut diamond ring was on my finger, my mind fast forwarded to what I pictured our life would be like together, and my heart felt full; I was ready to be his wife, and in due time, a mother to some beautiful chocolate babies.

For the next few months, we spent time together, alternating from the Bronx, Alexandria, and Atlanta. Finally, the travels came to an end when I officially moved. On the 26th of September 2015, I was on a one-way flight from LaGuardia Airport in New York City to Hartsfield-Jackson in Atlanta, Georgia. However, I was to arrive at a beautiful house that wouldn't feel like home.

For the first few weeks, while at the house, something new was constantly being delivered. A new couch one day, a painting or new appliance another day; yet I had not been a part of picking any of it. Also, I was in a new city where we had to drive every-where. I really began to miss not only my MetroCard, but also my mother, my friends, and everything that came with being in New York City.

At first, I figured it was just an adjustment and was hopeful things would get better with time. But I felt sad every day and living together wasn't as great as I had thought it would be.

I expressed how I felt left out; however, it was not received well. Discussions turned into verbal matches, then week-long silent treatments. Over the next few months, I lost close to twenty pounds; going from a slim–fit to looking extremely thin and frail. I had daily migraines, falling asleep was a challenge, and when I would finally get some rest, I would be awakened from a deep sleep by the very man I had entrusted with my heart; helping him-self to my body without my consent.

Instinctively, I would slap his hand away. Nevertheless, he would continue, but with more force; placing his body on top of mine and pleasuring himself. After the first few times, I stopped fighting him off.

With each passing day, my will to live became weaker and weaker, and my mind would drift elsewhere; thinking about work and what I needed to get done, instead of what was happening at that moment.

It was then that my hair started to fall out.

What was once a healthy head of natural hair was now dry, brittle, and all over the bathroom sink every time I combed it.

Looking into the mirror, I would just stare and ask myself, "How did I get here?"

I needed to figure it out and plan an exit strategy QUICKLY because, at the pace things were going, I was on an express train to my deathbed. I lived with an overwhelming sense of embarrassment for months when I recognized that I had made a mistake in accepting this marriage proposal.

To distract my mind, I did what I do best. I went to work. Although I am not a morning person, I went to work early, stayed late and even got another job so that I could be 'busy.' On average I was working 80+ hours per week. One evening, I got back to the house, and he says to me, "Your other dude must be a happy man with all that time you spend with him."

I replied, "I would be happy to if that man existed." I thought to myself, *FOOL! If you don't shut the entire hell up with this bullshit!* At the same time, the need to explain anything to him was in the toilet. If he wanted to believe I was being unfaithful, I did absolutely nothing to reassure him otherwise.

Truthfully, it was amusing that he was jealous and fabricated some drawn out story about my being with another man. I even joined in and started to fantasize about this imaginary man. I thought about him daily and gave him qualities and identified values that I needed in a life partner.

I found myself thinking A LOT.

Looking back, majoring in social work in undergrad was the beginning of my journey to deep self-reflection and being in tune with my feelings. I had to be honest with where I was; *yes, I felt embarrassed.* However, I can't and shouldn't stay angry with myself just because of one decision.

Undergrad was the first time I participated in therapy. For a long time, my purpose had been tied to being present and helpful to everyone around me. In order to be helpful, I had to be in a good space first. Therapy helped me in my early career as a social worker, making me aware that I had faith, and that I could get back to a space where I radiated goddess vibes of elegance, grace, and strength. Only this time, it would be from the inside. I needed to get better and be better for me.

I was buying groceries at the farmers market one day, and as I was waiting to check out, a woman behind me said to me, "You have a good grade of hair. If my hair was like that, I wouldn't need a relaxer."

If I had a nickel for every time I have been told this, I would be **very** wealthy. Words are powerful, and what we say out loud have conscious and subconscious meaning. I asked the woman what she meant by 'good grade of hair,' and her response was, "You know, your hair is not nappy like mine."

In my mind, I was thinking *if you only knew what my hair looks like if I don't take care of it.*

I have learned to embrace my hair the way it is at every stage of my natural hair journey, but most importantly, I focus on the health of my mind. I had to challenge what I have been taught about my hair and how it looks to focus on what I really feel about myself and how I present myself to the world unapologetically.

"Don't touch my hair when it's the feelings I wear."
-Solange

As more hair was falling out, I gelled down what was still attached to my scalp into a low bun and prepared to attend my younger sister's wedding on June 30, 2016.

On that day, it was the happiest I had felt in months! We drove to Birmingham, Alabama, and it was the first time that I had seen my parents and my siblings in one space since I had moved to Atlanta the previous year. My sister and her new husband radiated so much love on that day; it was a reminder that the love and support I needed in my life were real and the relationship that I was in *was not it*.

The days following the wedding, I quietly began to look for places to live, and on July 14th, I signed the lease to my new apartment, my hand trembling as I paid my deposit. It was like my body was moving and making decisions that I should have made months prior. I felt a sense of relief that I would soon have a place to call home. I ended the engagement, moved out on August 24th, and have been thriving since!

Thriving emotionally, I have taken the time to heal my heart and shed the weight of expectations of where I should be at this stage of my life as a single woman, with no children or a husband. Thriving physically, as I have gained all the weight I initially lost, plus a little extra, and my hair is the healthiest it has ever been.

I have learned through my faith and in therapy, that obstacles build posture; and this experience, although challenging, has served me well in recognizing what will not work for me.

The bigger my afro gets, the more people want to touch it. I am the lady random people walk up to with arms and hands extended, reaching out to touch my hair.

I understand being curious; however, think twice before you walk up to a melanated beauty and put your hands on her hair. The universal response is typically a side-eye, with tons of questions running through her mind like, *"Did they just touch my hair?" "Are their hands even clean?" "Are you for real right now?"*

Deciding to stop chemically straightening your hair is the first step; as you start to shed the straight hair and embrace the kinky, curly coils that blossom from your scalp, you will be received differently in all areas of your life.

For me, the areas that challenged me the most were in my career, my love life, and growing into my womanhood.

When I started working in the social work field in June 2009, all my hair was natural at this point, and I struggled with how I would wear my hair to work because I wanted to look 'professional.' My go-to style at the time was a handful of gel, brushing my hair down into a low bun and keeping that style for the week. Then, after the probation period was over, I would wear my hair brushed back, but instead of the bun, I would rock my puff.

The first time I wore a puff to work, I was so nervous!

I was working as a case manager at a preventive service agency in Harlem. When I interviewed for the job, attire was emphasized as business casual as my role included going out into the community. There was an extensive part of the discussion that included hair; I remember being told to look neat.

Let's pause here. What exactly is 'neat'?

For naturals, which include loose hair (afros), locs, sister locs, and braids, this is a huge topic of discussion that has made it to news station segments, magazine articles, and videos on social media platforms. Are you really trying to say that these kinky curls and coils that grow from my scalp, and defy gravity, are not 'neat'?

Children have been suspended for wearing their hair, whether in locs, braids, braids with beads, or their afros and penalized for not meeting the institution's dress code, being told that their hairstyle is a distraction to the academic setting. The message that is delivered is that as people from the African diaspora, our hair does not meet the Eurocentric standard of what is considered beautiful or appropriate in educational settings and corporate America.

Singling out a person about their hair can be shaming, isolating, and can even trigger symptoms of anxiety and depression. Black clients I have worked with in therapy have asked questions that include, but are not limited to, "Are my braids work appropriate?" "Are my locs too much for this interview?" and "Should I just get a wig or a weave so that my hair looks presentable?"

Self-esteem is a person's emotional assessment of how they view themselves. Hair-esteem is similar, in that it's a person's emotional assessment of how they view their hair. Both can be skewed, based on life experiences such as trauma, family perception, the media, and ethnicity within the African diaspora.

Hair typing is a spectrum that identifies hair from straight to kinky curls/coils. What I learned about my natural hair is that it's not all one texture; on my left side, my hair has a looser curl pattern. On the right side, my hair has tight kinky coils and in between it just depends on the day.

I have encountered naturals who have either done the big chop or are gradually cutting their relaxed hair as they transition back to natural hair, who would often ask what hair products I use or even comment on my hair texture.

When I interviewed for my most recent position as a therapist in an outpatient mental health clinic, I wore my hair in a twist out and was offered the job!

Boom

Before the interview, I had to think about how I am presenting myself as it relates to my career. I love my natural hair and getting into an emotional space where I can confidently walk into a professional setting and be my true *self* was a huge step! As a therapist, it was hypocritical to teach people how to cope with symptoms and how to be authentic in all areas of their lives when I wasn't doing the same.

Today I proudly wear my natural hair to work regularly and teach anyone that is willing to listen how to shift their mindset about natural hair.

As a result of my love for natural hair and behavioral health, *Your Natural Hairapist* (YNH) was created.

YNH's mission is to support black women in gaining the confidence to overcome emotional barriers to obtain outward beauty. The purpose is to teach women through the use of webinars, events, and consultation/coaching to feel less self-conscious and more confident about every stage of their natural hair journey.

YNH is a social platform to highlight the beauty of being natural, as well as addressing the real-life psychosocial stressors that black women face as they transition and maintain their natural hair.

When I think of who I am as a woman, and how I made it to where I am at this very moment, a lot of it had to do with external factors. All of my experiences, positive and character-building have twisted, tied, and pulled me in directions that had the potential to break and sink the human spirit. My faith and personal journey in therapy have been the driving force in healing from the past, teaching me to be mindful of taking care of myself, and being in tune with how I feel when I feel it.

My past hair loss experience was more than just my hair falling out; the stress that was in my body disrupted the flow of systems that promote healthy living.

For you, it may not be stress like it was for me. It may be a medical condition, poor diet, or just not knowing what to do with your hair. In your natural hair journey, YNH's mission is to help you feel empowered to embrace the beauty that is already within you. We live in an age where social media and the internet have a vast variety of resources available at our fingertips.

However, all information is not useful, and this is where discernment kicks in. Being knowledgeable about the ingredients of hair products has been the single most important thing that I have learned in my journey to holistic health as it relates to my body and the internal/external care of my hair.

I had to learn what my hair likes, and when I found the right products, it made a huge difference in how I was able to care for my hair and how I felt wearing my hair natural.

Being cost effective is also helpful. **CurlBox**, a monthly subscription to hair products, has saved me so much money!

Ultimately, I am a firm believer that there is nothing a woman can't do in an amazing pair of heels.

...and slayed hair!

RAISING OURSELVES

By Catrece M. Davis, LCSW

"Who is Catrece Davis?" you ask.

You ask, "Who is Catrece Davis?"

I say a beautiful, educated, clinical social worker, mentor, mother, wife, friend, sister, and a believer in change, but I did not always feel this way. I was that lost little girl who felt so alone because of the lack of guidance and support from my mother

I think back on my life and the experiences I have gone through, some without a choice and some that were choices of my own, based on what I knew. I was conceived from an affair my mother had with my father while married to my sister and brother's father—my stepfather. I was not told about this difference and about not having the same father as my siblings until I was six or seven.

Timelines are not concrete because my life was so fast-paced and filled with drama! I am the youngest of three.

My mother had my sister at 15, my brother at 17, and me at 19. I know that's a lot of children... my mother was a teen mother with three children before age 20!

We left Arkansas, from my understanding, before I was one. We were so far from home with little support, and only my stepfather—who was in the military and stationed in California on Vandenberg Air Force Base—to rely on.

Things began to fall apart, in my eyes, when my stepfather decided to leave my mother and us. Fighting was a regular thing, and infidelity, drinking, and lack of concern for what we had going on was a consistent pattern in our home.

Mental illness was prevalent but was untreated as my mother self-medicated by drinking. I remember the day my stepfather left. He tried to leave, and my mother was trying to get him to stay. My siblings and I were crying in the driveway as he took his luggage out of the house; my mother is crying, he was yelling, and both of them were fighting.

Then, he drove off.

Although, in reality, he was not my biological father, he was the only father I knew at that time. We were told he left for another woman, whom he did marry and have two more children with, in addition to raising her son from a previous relationship.

This whole situation took our lives—my mother's, my siblings', and mine—on a spiraling downward cycle. These experiences left my mom empty and broken with the inability to love herself, or us, in a way that was needed.

Depression was real but masked by drinking.

My mother blamed everyone else and would take her anger out on us. I have been whipped with extension cords, shoes, belts, switches, whatever she could grab.

I was called "bitch," a lot. This became the pet name she called my sister and me... and still does, if I open the door too wide or engage too much.

We did have to move off base, as I remember, IMMEDIATELY! We moved to this rundown apartment complex called Kalani Village in Lompoc, California. My mother did all she could because she had been working on base in the commissary at the time. I have few memories there.

One of the memories was the time my mother was about to whip me after my brother caught me behind the trash can with a boy from the apartment complex (they say I was trying to have sex or give oral sex, I believe).

Once he caught us, my brother ran back to the apartment and told my mother. She was trying to get to me, so I ran and hid under the bed and continued to scream because I did not want what she was about to give. I knew I had done something bad but did not know what I was doing. I continued to scream so loud that a neighbor called the police. My mother was upset with the neighbors, and she went on a rant about someone calling on her.

The police wanted to see me to make sure I was okay. Once they did so, my mother was given a warning, and the whole whipping ordeal was over. Thank God for that neighbor, because I know the situation would have turned out differently that night had she not been interrupted.

Not too long before the whole incident, I had been violated by an old white man living in the apartment complex. Because my mother had to work, or she was in the apartment doing her own thing, we were able to roam around the complex and I was always trying to keep up with my siblings.

On this day, the man lured my sister and me into his apartment with the promise of candy. I remember being close to him as he sat and massaged my private area with his hand in my panties while talking to me. Although I don't remember being penetrated, the vivid memory of his touching me and looking at me while he did it is still a clear picture in my head.

All this happened at approximately five years old.

My sister and I never talked about it, and we still have not. I never told anyone and did not tell my mother until I was an adult when we were discussing the past. My mother did eventually get us out of there, and though things were not all back together, she was able to move us into a better situation.

Transitions continued in my life. We had a period of peace until my mother decided to go back for "that" visit to Arkansas. I thought we were going to visit my great-grandmother and other family members. But, now that I think about it, I think this visit was for her to reconnect with my father now that she wasn't married to my stepfather anymore. In hindsight, I do believe my mother and father had that soul-tie type relationship.

My mother took me off by myself and explained that I would be meeting someone, not yet telling me it would be my real father. Then, the grand introduction happened... he spoke, I spoke, but I did not say much more because I did not know how to feel. I don't remember much, other than I told my siblings once I returned. Again, until that point, I had only known my siblings' father as my "real" father. I did not know how to feel.

When we went home, he followed.

Here we go again!

My mother brought my father back to California with us, and once again our lives were in turmoil because he caused so much havoc; my mother lost jobs because *he* would get caught cheating at a job *she* helped him get. They would fight (on the job), and ultimately, she would lose her job.

Drugs and needles were introduced into my life when I found a bag of needles in the garage and asked what they were for. They partied, and then they would fight. He would be us for nothing.

Like the time I laid my new coat down to play with other kids while waiting for the teacher to come and open the door. He drove by, and the next thing I knew I was being questioned about my new coat. He then took his belt off and whipped me in front of my entire class.

I remember him hollering at me about my new coat and what would happen to me if I did it again. I also remember running into my class, kids explaining to my teacher what happened, and my retreating under the table because of embarrassment and shame. I remember my teacher trying to coerce me to come out because I would NOT.

How could I face my peers?

My mother did nothing about his actions and just allowed him to come in and take over. Doing as he pleased and beating us when he chose. My father beat the hell out of my mother, and then they would rekindle the flame. The honeymoon period always came around. Situation after situation!

The cycle was vicious! Just too much!

Domestic violence was a daily occurrence, or at least it seemed to be daily. I remember seeing my father whip my mother with a water hose in our backyard, while we were looking out the patio window—scared—knowing that we could not do anything because we didn't want to get it; only to see them intimately engaging the next day.

When I walked into her room to let her know I was home, I was so mad at her after I had walked in on them because she had put him out. "Where *was my mother?*" I asked myself. Did she care about us at all?

She had lost herself!

Back then my mother focused solely on herself, the men in her life, working, drinking, and partying. We were not her main priority, or even second or third. At least how I felt at that time. We would be left at other people's homes for days. My father did eventually leave my mother, which I was glad about. But, I believe that is when my mother's depressive symptoms, reckless behavior, and drinking worsened.

Combing my own hair, dressing myself, feeding myself, getting my stuff together, getting to school without the assistance of my mother was a regular thing. I never knew if my mother would be home or not.

When I look back on things now, I see that my mother was doing the best that she could with the tools she was given.

See, my mother had lost her mother when she was only two years old. Her mother died two weeks after having my uncle due to birthing complications. So, my mother had been raised by her grandmother. I remember her telling me a story about when she was about to move to California with my stepfather, and how she begged my great-grandmother not to make her go as my stepfather was already beating her.

But, because my great-grandmother was old school, she believed that my mother should go and be with her children's father and her husband.

My mother was consistent with working, having a man, and drinking and kicking it. Love was never expressed in our home and good times were few and far between (my mother still struggles to tell me that she loves me to this day).

I say this not to hurt my mother, but to say that going through this process called life without the basic supports of either my mother or father created a hole in me that has taken years to fix, or, shall I say, fixed enough to survive. I do have a better understanding now, knowing that my mother had a problematic childhood, and generationally there were issues passed down to her.

My mother never got help for all her issues and untreated mental illness (depression/PTSD and grief from the loss of her mother). Substance abuse (alcohol) was her way of trying to numb herself from the pain she had experienced in life. Now that I know some of the things that my mother has gone through, I make a practice of being less judgmental of her and the choices she made to survive in what was a very lonely world for her.

She wanted to be loved, too.

Yes, I was forced to make decisions for myself without a choice. The lack of support I received taught me to be strong, to protect myself, and not to depend on anyone. That thought process also caused some struggles that I could have avoided as a teen if I hadn't always tried to handle things on my own.

When will the roller coaster stop!? My mother could not raise us anymore, and situations worsened to the point that my mother had to make the decision to send us away to live with our great grandmother back in Arkansas. I was approximately ten, I believe, and abandoned. *She is so selfish. I hate her. She chose herself over her children... again. She chose alcohol over her children... again. She chose men over her children... again.*

I was blaming her and not realizing that by sending us away, she was trying to love us in the best way she knew how. Living in Arkansas with my great-grandmother was one of the only times in my life I remember being nurtured, taken care of, loved, and safe. I struggled to receive what was offered by my great grandmother because, no matter how much love my great-grandmother tried to show me, I wanted my mama.

There was one instance where my stepfather came back in the picture while we still lived with my great grandmother. We were all "afforded" the opportunity to come live with him and his family. My brother and I decided to go, leaving my sister behind. That was six months of blur!

I remember losing my virginity to my stepbrother, his son, at approximately age 12... yeah, that's right, because I was in the 7th grade. My stepbrother was 15 or 16 at the time. I was coerced. It started with him playfully touching me to see how far he could go. Then he began to become more physical (groping), then penetration with his hands, ultimately leading to full-on sexual intercourse.

This happened over a span of days.

As I look at it now, he took advantage of me and for years I thought it was my fault because I was "fast," but he was the elder of the two, and he was the one who initiated the behaviors preceding sex. But, back then I consented, which caused me to rationalize it as being okay. I didn't know any better, and no one told me it was *not* okay.

I remember becoming increasingly promiscuous, failing school, and wanting to go back to my great-grandmother.

My step-mother was also exposing me to things I should not have seen, and she was not a healthy role model for me. She would take me to the convenience store with her at night while she worked, and for several nights in a row, a man would sit in the parking lot and jack off in his car—visibly! She would encourage me to look and watch. I did tell my father that this was happening, and soon after that, they sent me back to Arkansas with my great grandmother.

Obviously, as a child, I was under-parented; a parentified child as I've learned through educating myself. Feelings of abandonment, shame, loneliness, confusion, despair, guilt, and low self-worth were all twirling around in my head. Thoughts turned to behaviors, and behaviors turned into habits that took me a long time to break.

It was easy for me to detach because of how I had been brought up. Protecting myself, so I thought, to prevent getting close enough to allow anyone to hurt me.

The road I took once I returned from my stepfather's house was a treacherous one. No one cared anyway, or at least that was my thought at that period in my life. Habitual thoughts in my head of confusion, impulsivity, not caring, and self-destruction were upon me! I just didn't give a fuck—literally!

When I think back, I can see how I treated myself so badly. Again, I saw too much as a child! The choices my mother made, I found myself making by misusing my body, living life recklessly, and not giving a damn about my future. Choices my mother made affected the entire structure of our family.

And, things got worse before getting better.

My uncle and grandmother found out that I was having sex after my cousin contacted them and let them know that I must have had someone over while babysitting because the boy had left a "present" in their bed. My uncle made me strip and whipped me for what seemed like hours. I was shamed once again, being 15, and having to take my clothes off in front of my uncle. As he whipped me, I flailed around trying to take the pain.

My grandmother finally came in and told him to stop! I was placed on punishment for three to four months.

As a teen, I did not care about my future. I continued promiscuity without thought, getting pregnant at 15, and forcefully punching my stomach daily, for weeks, until it was no more! I did not want to be 15 and pregnant like my mother.
I couldn't take care of a baby!

I had nothing to give at that time.

My great grandmother put me on a Greyhound bus to California a few months later because she could not handle me anymore. I think I just wanted my mother at the time and thought things had to be better than here. Shit got worse, but also better in the sense that I did learn skills I used to survive my journey.

I continued to make negative choices, exhibit impulsiveness, and have low self-esteem. Though my mother was finally present, in the sense that we were living under the same roof, she was still doing the same things: men, work, and drinking.

So many things happened in that three-year period: moving from Arkansas to Los Angeles, failing school, getting caught on campus drunk, skipping daily, running away, attempting suicide (took a bottle of tetracycline), and ultimately dropping out of high school. Two positives that did come out of the situation were learning how to swim and eventually becoming a lifeguard for the city of Los Angeles and meeting my husband (Marcus).

The pool was my safe haven! I spent countless hours at the pool trying to stay out of trouble, but the impulsive *me* did not stay settled long!

At 18, I was arrested for shoplifting with my roommate. I was 18 with an arrest record, no high school diploma, and little to fall back on, other than my man and the lifeguarding job I had. So, one of the very first lessons I learned from this incident was not to take things that did not belong to me (something I probably should have learned earlier but didn't). Once I got out, I promised myself that I would not do anything else that could cause me to go back to jail and lose my freedom.

Those were the worst four days —yes, FOUR days—of my life; hands down.

My mother had moved back to Arkansas by that time because my great grandmother had become ill. I decided to stay in California when my mother offered for me to return to Arkansas with her. I knew nothing was there for me, in Arkansas, and my mother had shown me she wasn't going to change.

That was the best decision of my LIFE!

My journey has been a learning process, a healing process, and a growth process, with still so much more work to do. I don't blame my mother for things I did once I knew better, because they were my choices. I made my journey harder, initially. I was never afraid to try new things—both good and bad—but, once I got tired of bumping my head, I began to listen, starting with influential people in my life whom God had strategically placed there for me. I thank God every day for His blessings!

I never had that connection or bond that most little girls desire to have with their mother. She just was not emotionally available. Like she said, "I did all I could do." I have always desired a relationship with my mother and have tried to mend it, but I always get hurt, so I have learned to love from a distance.

In my later years, I have been more empathetic to her situation. I couldn't imagine having three children by 19-years-old, dependent on my husband, and living far away from my family.

As I grew and educated myself, I knew that what my mother was going through was deeper than us. She suffered from child sexual abuse, the death of her mother, domestic violence, substance abuse, relational issues, disconnection from her children, poor choice-making, generational trauma, and untreated mental health issues.

The experiences I have been through have shaped how I engage with my daughters. I did not want them to ever feel or experience the things I did. My experiences have guided me toward my passions for helping others, specifically teen girls. I think that was the stage in my life that I felt the most lost, vulnerable, and alone. I lost control because I did not care, so I thought. I felt no one understood me and what I needed.

I needed my mama!

I had to soul search and start looking at my own actions, instead of blaming my mother for all that had happened in my life. So, I began surrounding myself with others who motivated me to begin the process of moving forward to becoming a better me.

Somewhere along the line, I realized that if I wanted different, I had to act, think, and go about things differently. I was going to have to stop living in my past and begin working towards my future. Once I accomplished one thing, I wanted to accomplish others. Social work was not a choice for me. It is me; the only thing I could come up with that I love so much I would do it for free.

Still, my life did not change overnight. In fact, I continue to work on me daily. I think back to my teen years and how thankful I am for the two skills that kept me going during that time—typing and swimming. I learned both those skills during my short-lived time in the regular high school setting. They literally saved my life because I was always able to get a job.

But, without that high school diploma, my job selection was limited. I was 19 and living with my husband when I decided to go back to school to get my diploma. My mother had moved back to Arkansas and then on to Chicago after that. I was in California just living—no, sinking, really—but trying to make it. Marcus and I were roughing it, though he did not have to; he had his mother and her support if he needed to go back home, but he decided to stay with me.

At first, this did not sit well with his mother, but I did eventually win her over. He was my first supporter other than my great grandmother as I see it. He was there for me and did not *have* to be.

We did have rough times, but my husband would always encourage me to go for it whenever it came to improving myself. My old high school principal contacted me out of the blue and explained the school would be holding night classes for people who wanted to return to get their diploma.

Despite still making financial and relationship mistakes, I did know that going back to school was needed for me to grow.

So, I started.

During that time, my supporters were my husband, his mother, my high school principal, and my favorite teacher to this day, Mr. Olivadoti, known affectionately as "Mr. O." Previously, I despised this man and would argue, cuss him out, and walk out of class while enrolled in regular continuation (alternative learning environment). However, once I was in night school, I saw a different Mr. O. It was just the two of us on most nights because all the classes I had to make up were with him.

He took his time and was not the same teacher I encountered when I was with my peers and acting out for a laugh. During night school, Mr. O. knew I was serious and that this time I would finish. He, as well as my principal, Mrs. Kamora, would drive me home at night to help; they allowed me to be vulnerable and accept their support because of their kindness and genuine concern about my life and outcomes.

On the day of my graduation, the only two who were there specifically for me was my husband and my homegirl Tracy. No one in my immediate family attended. Not my mother, siblings, or father. Still, I was so proud of myself that day!

Step one completed!

I can remember when they called my name, and Marcus began to scream from the stands, as I walked up to receive my diploma. That is how he continued to congratulate me throughout my years in college. I desired for my mother to be at one of my graduations, which did happen later when I received my bachelor's degree.

There were periods of both progress and decline even after I graduated from college. I knew social work was it for me as a career, and that the field I had chosen to invest my life in was a field that would also allow me to heal myself by giving to others.

Getting married, having children, having a career in place, making money, and moving forward allowed me to think that things were good and finally coming together. Little did I know that the past traumas in my life were always lurking.

I recently began therapy myself to truly heal and be whole. Resiliency and perseverance are two things that I think helped me get through to this point.

And, the things I have learned are:

1. My past is my past.
2. Choices determine the direction of my life.
3. Hard work does pay off.
4. Believing in self and having healthy self-esteem is essential to healing.,
5. Letting go of things that hurt you is best.
6. Forgive for yourself, and not for others.
7. Step out on faith and believe in yourself.
8. Never be afraid of change.

These are all things I took with me once I moved back to Arkansas from California to begin my higher education journey and entry into the social work field. My life has changed drastically over the years. So many life lessons learned, both by listening to others and, yes, also the hard way.

I always knew there had to be more, though, and that intuition, that gut feeling was right. So many pitfalls, hurdles, and changes in my life happened while on this journey to find wholeness. The roles are still skewed when it comes to my mother and me, but I have learned to let her live her life as I am learning to live mine without regret.

I was my mother's emotional support while witnessing her alcoholism and depression increase. I learned that I could not take on my mother's problems and that in order to heal, I had to do what was best for me without so much focus on her.

Having to take care of myself has been a process that has gone on for 46 years. I have had to humble myself and surrender to things I could not change. I have accomplished many things I did not think I could; however, believing in myself, and taking a chance on me, in spite of my fucked-up past, has changed my life for the better. The effects of childhood trauma did not resonate with me until my therapist began to help me see that raising myself truly impacted me.

Through telling my story, I hope to help others understand and believe that old cliché "Your past does not determine your future despite the hand you have been dealt!"

I hope readers can relate to the experiences I've shared about my life and my journey of survival to living a healthier, happier, more meaningful life—changing myself and working on me, both inside and out. I want readers to finish my chapter having a better understanding of a parentified child, and how I navigated through with the understanding that if I wanted something to change in my life, I would have to be the initiator.

Finally, I would like to bring to light to how generational trauma and lack of support from a parent can have a great impact on the African American child. Often issues are not addressed and mental health challenges go untreated.

In Black community there are so many barriers to having a healthy mind. Without resolution, patterns are passed down from one generation to the next. The cycle continues when there is no change in mindset.

Trauma is a part of me but does not rule me. I learned that in therapy.

Post-traumatic growth. Not damaged goods!

TEK CYEAR A DE ROOT

By Victoria Y. Miller, MS

Mus tek cyear a de root fa heal da tree is a Gullah proverb that translates to, you must take care of the root in order to heal the tree. This saying is rich in truth and provides the framework for the helping professional. These words are steeped into the history of my Gullah, or Geechee, speaking people who originated from eighteenth and nineteenth century enslaved Africans from West and Central Africa; landing on the Sea Islands off the coasts of the Carolinas, Georgia, and Florida.

I live my life by this philosophy through my work and relationships. If one cannot locate and repair the damages imposed by the environment from which the tree grew, the inner bark is surely to become scarred, broken, attract disease, and unable to heal over time.

I was born and raised in Charleston, South Carolina; a place that I am proud to claim, but also one steeped in history and shame. As a dark-skinned black girl growing up in the South from a low-income household, I was raised by parents who had less than a high school education.

Therefore, I am all too familiar with the internal, and external, hardships and struggles that can be present in the family, as well as the community. It was there that I discovered the true meaning of not having a "pot to piss in or a window to throw it out of." It was there that I also discovered my love for *"white people shit."*

The first time I found out about white people shit, I was in elementary school. The television was often my babysitter because my mother and stepfather worked full-time jobs to support the household. I watched shows with predominately white cast members; such as Bay Watch, Beverly Hills 90210, and almost the entire TGIF weekly broadcast on ABC.

The days with my grandmother and great aunt, my babysitters, were spent watching soap operas like, *The Young and the Restless*, *As the World Turns*, *Passions*, *Days of Our Lives*, and whatever other soap opera dominated the television screen during that time.

The Winter and Summer Olympic games of the 90s introduced me to the phrase "white people shit." I remember watching figure skating and gymnastic competitions showcasing the talents of Tara Lipinski, Michelle Kwan, Oksana Baiul, Dominique Dawes, and the magnificent seven to name a few. I thought to myself *I want to be them.*

I remember telling my mother how much I wanted to be an ice skater and work the balance beams. She gave me a perplexed look, and then with a stern voice exclaimed, *"O gal, please. That's white people shit,"* followed by a nervous laugh.

Not fully understanding what she meant, a few days later, I inquired again while we drove past a center for gymnastics. Without hesitation, she said, *"You got money for that? Gal, you have to have money to do that type of thing."*

I was defeated, but my young impressionable mind finally understood what she meant by "white people shit."

After that day, I never shared these desires again.

One day, while my mother and grandmother went on their Saturday morning garage sale excursion to the middle-class neighborhoods, my mother found a pair of Fisher Price "Grow With Me" beginner roller skates. The skates were blue and yellow with orange wheels, had three adjustment settings for levels of advancement, and came with matching elbow and knee pads for added protection.

These skates were hideous but became one of my favorite childhood toys. I loved those skates so much, that I often found myself in trouble for trying to skate with them around the house after the street lights illuminated our block; indicating the time for me, my friends, and my cousins to depart to our homes in the Emanuel Methodist Episcopal (EME) apartments, which we affectionately called *The Project*.

I was a natural.

It did not take very long for me to graduate from my beginner skates to the skates at the Hot Wheels Skating Rink, where my friends and family members often gathered on the weekend to show off the latest moves, stalk our neighborhood crush, and get away from the humdrum of everyday life. I often wonder how different my life would be if I had never heard the phrase "white people shit."

Could I have been the next Mabel Fairbanks or Surya Bonaly? If given the opportunity, could my name have been mentioned with the greats of the new millennium such as Gabrielle Douglas or Simone Biles?

What I learned at that tender development stage is that only white people were afforded the best things in life, and my black ass was left with whatever those white folks sold in their front yards on Saturday mornings. I found myself infatuated, mesmerized, consumed, and overly obsessed with "white people shit." I wanted to be a white woman. Dare I say it? I wanted her skin tone and I wanted her hair; I wanted to talk, walk, dress, and act like her.

Being white seemed to be a hell of a lot better than being black. Every toy commercial I saw showcased white children happily playing with toys I could only dream of having, but because I was not white, I could not afford them. It was also embedded in me at a young age that toys with the same hue as me were only good enough to be displayed in the corner of the screen, in a circle small enough to see that there were different shades of the same doll available, at the very end of the commercial. I questioned how I could be more involved in "white people shit" without being white.

Not receiving any support from home, I came up with the idea that if I surrounded myself with white people, I would soon be doing *white people shit* like Lisa Turtle on *Saved by the Bell*. I began to view shows like *The Cosby Show* and *A Different World* as the blueprint to entering my fantasy white world instead of gaining the perspective that "white people shit" was not limited to just white people.

My senior year in high school, I visited the guidance counselor to discuss plans for graduation and beyond. For the first time, my love for education reawakened thanks to this fair skinned, blonde haired, blue eyed school employee. We discussed the college admission process, and I was provided with several books and resources to get me started. However, I was unclear on how I would pay for my education and spent many sleepless nights thinking I was in over my head. There was no way a poor black girl like me could pay for college or gain acceptance. I turned to my mother for help, but her response, *"O gal, please. What you need to go to more school for? You can get a good job here."*

My mother's idea of a good job was making enough to pay the bills and make it to the next paycheck. It was all she knew, but I knew better. I had the blueprint to living a better life ingrained in my subconscious. And, although there were often talks of the importance of money, what was lacking from the conversation was how to get it... and keep it.

Education was not a top priority in my household, either. I was an Honor Roll student, and had received several academic awards; however, as time passed, the awards and recognition were seldom celebrated in my home. I recall a time I won a literary award at Murray LaSaine Elementary School. I was so very proud of this achievement. I had written a creative short story based on my favorite food, chocolate. There was an award ceremony held for the winners.

I did not attend.

What was the reason you ask?

"O gal, please. I don't have time for that. I have to work. You will be alright," was the explanation my mother gave. With my head held low, I told my teacher the next day that I was not able to attend because my mother was sick. I was ashamed. I was not lectured on the importance of education, or praised for my achievements; therefore, I eventually traded in my high academic standing to just fit in and become an average student, working after school to help pay the bills. After all, good grades and academic honors were not

getting me closer to my dreams of being a materialistically rich, worthy of praise, white woman.

Eventually, a light bulb went off, and I concluded that college was my only way out. Despite my mother's best efforts to dissuade me from my educational pursuits, I was accepted to Columbia College in Columbia, South Carolina. I later transferred to and graduated from, the University of South Carolina, just a few blocks away.

My mother helped me the best she could to get money for tuition, by asking for loans from the bank and extended family members who had previously sent their children to college, but to no avail. Having gotten pregnant in high school, my mother's education had ended, and thus, she was ill-equipped to help me pursue advanced education and had no idea how to guide me in the right direction. I decided that if this was something I wanted, I would have to figure it out on my own. For my sweet mother did not understand my love for "white people shit."

College opened my eyes to a whole new perspective on the subject. Growing up in the quaint town of James Island, there was not much diversity. My world was black and white. In college, my black peers were no longer of the same lower class as me; they were living my white dreams. They had supportive parents who understood the importance of obtaining a good education. They drove nice cars, wore nice clothes, spoke proper English, and were intelligent.

This was a cultural shock to me!

My friends were the Huxtables, descendants of Hillman College, and closely familiar with the 90210 ZIP Code.

Unfortunately, my financial situation did not allow me to enjoy the freedom that came with becoming a blossoming adult woman in a higher education institution. I often found myself working two jobs to help pay my tuition and living expenses, while also sending money home to my financially crippled family.

Of course, I have fond memories of my college experience, but they are not free of guilt. Because I often had to send money home to help my parents keep their heads above water, while I was struggling to stay afloat, I began to despise "white people shit."

My mother was right. Who was I to think I could ever have an American dream that was never meant for me or people who looked like me?

Presently, I am a non-commissioned officer in the United States Army, and a Marriage and Family Therapy PhD candidate. I often describe myself as a versatile and self-motivated scholar-practitioner dedicated to the academic, personal, and professional advancement of myself and others. Furthermore, I rely on my past experiences and newfound knowledge to guide my interactions and work with others. I have been able to thrive, despite the odds against me.

However, I have not always been this way.

My mother's perspective on subjects such as education has had lasting effects. Oftentimes, I found myself feeling as though my accomplishments just weren't good enough. Therefore, I found little fulfillment in my achievements, and was on a constant search for validation in various aspects of my life such as relationships, work, career, and academia; merely escaped undergraduate school with a 2.3 GPA and the belief that I was unworthy of achieving my dreams.

Where did my mother's attitude that only white people were afforded to live, work, and play in luxury come from? Was this taught, learned, or inherited behavior?

I have a praying grandmother. My grandmother, Anna Mae Jenkins, was one of eleven children and had eight girls of her own. She attended school in a one-room shack, but education did not continue any further than that.

Born in 1937, she witnessed and experienced the ramifications of war, racism, discrimination, and overall oppression of the African American people. My grandmother was taught to survive; a lesson she taught her children that has been passed down through generations. But how does one turn negative adaptive behaviors into positive ones?

> *"You may not control all the events that happen to you,*
> *but you can decide not to be reduced by them."*
> -Maya Angelou[1]

Imagine feeling like a stranger in your own home. Feeling as though you must be deaf, blind, and dumb to the systematic oppression that has crippled you and those that look like you because that's the way it has always been.

This is the reality of the African American.

African Americans have been institutionally oppressed by those who have become desensitized by the very system they built to demean, shame, victimize, and dehumanize a person of color.

So, what does this mean for the black experience?

---

[1] Letter to my Daughter; 2008

Yes, we've made notable strides in medical, social, literary, political, cultural, and astrological fields; however, there is still so much work to do in our advancement of mental health.

I know there may be many, both within and outside the community, that ask the question *"If we have come so far, how are we still an oppressed people?"* The answer? Historical trauma.

We must understand how the baggage of internalized trauma has manifested into our external realities.

Trauma

Those who experience trauma, or a deeply disturbing experience, are often left mentally and physically debilitated, and diagnosed with trauma-and stressor-related disorders.

Intergenerational effect of trauma on minority groups has been addressed in previous studies as posttraumatic slave syndrome, second-generation trauma, historical trauma, and transgenerational transmission of trauma.

It is theorized that trauma in a community has long-standing effects that can be passed on through generations. The African American community has endured much historical trauma stemming from racism and discrimination. Yet, the Diagnostic and Statistical Manual of Mental Disorders does not take intergenerational into account when outlining the criteria for post-traumatic stress disorder (PTSD); a traumatic disorder that has been found to be more prevalent among the black community, with a national average of one in ten becoming traumatized in their lifetime.

Other findings have revealed that African Americans are pre-disposed to heightened stress as a result of historical traumas they have experienced, actual and perceived racial discrimination have been found to negatively affect mental and physical health, and racial minority military personnel have been found to have a higher likelihood of receiving a diagnosis of PTSD.

Historical Trauma

What is historical trauma, and what does it have to do with the current state of black mental health? What are the causes and how does one know when they, or their community, have been impacted? Historical trauma is an emotional wound that is carried from one generation to the next.

Think Erykah Badu's "Bag Lady."

The song refers to the emotional baggage a woman is carrying that is preventing her from forming a new relationship. This damage can stem from a relationship or something deeper; something she may have been predisposed to subconsciously. If I were to give myself the diagnosis of historical trauma, I might look into the following symptoms: depression, anxiety, loss of sleep, violence, and suicide, substance abuse, fear and distrust, discomfort around white people, loss of concentration, isolation, anger, and shame. Like Ms. Badu so eloquently put it, *"One day all them bags gone get in your way."*

Awareness is the first step to change.

I became aware that my thoughts and beliefs guided my behavior. It was not until I sought professional help, that I accepted this reality and took action toward change.

Sexual Abuse - Break de Cycle

The African American population has been exposed to generations of stressors caused by slavery, colonialism, racism, discrimination, and segregation. These stressors have resulted in violence, a distrust of authority, internalized racism, and different forms of abuse. One such abuse that is rarely talked about and remains a closeted issue is sexual abuse.

Sexual abuse in the African American community is the elephant in the room that desperately needs addressing. How many jokes have been made acceptable about the uncle who gets too familiar with the females of the family during family functions? Or, the overly friendly family friend everyone avoids, because of his over-sexualized sense of humor? When we ignore this deplorable behavior, it has lasting multigenerational effects.

60 percent of black girls experience sexual abuse by black men before the age of eighteen, and I am in that number. For me, I was molested by a family member while in the primary years of my education, and although I could not fully understand what I was experiencing, I do remember how I felt. The emotions eventually manifested themselves in confusion, anger, sexually acting out, violence, shame, guilt, distrust, low self-esteem, issues with authority figures, and anxiety.

More importantly, I remember how it felt to have my feelings dismissed by those I confided in and were supposed to protect me. Therefore, I often found myself looking for a savior in intimate relationships because unbeknown to me, the little girl inside of me was ever present; feeling like a victim.

Having carried this secret for years, I believed that revealing it would hurt the ones close to me and I just needed to be strong and bear this burden to protect them. However, as an adult with a daughter of my own, it is time that I no longer facilitate this dysfunction; preventing my daughter from repeating this pathology.

"In the year 1995, I decided to tell my mother that a family member often groped me when I was left alone with him. I was only nine, but I knew this was the end of my innocence. After writing a letter with as much detail as I could, I found my mother in the living room watching her favorite daytime series.

I decided to write a letter because it was the only way I knew how to express my feelings at the time. I handed her the letter, she read it, and then just looked at me.

As I opened my mouth, the words escaped my lips, but I could not hear them being spoken. I felt numb, ashamed. After what felt like an eternity, I heard my mother speak. 'He's just playing girl; he means no harm.' What I did not know at the time was that a similar situation happened to my mother who received the same response: 'He's just playing girl. He means no harm.'

I never spoke of it again, and the abuse continued."

Cases such as this are all too common. If this scenario made you uncomfortable, examine why. Do you know of a family friend, cousin, uncle, brother, or father that exhibits pedophilic or other perverse sexual behavior? What is the common consensus about this person?

As the old saying goes, *it takes a village to raise a child.* What will it take to protect that child? You cannot be free standing in your truth if you are still hiding.

Tek Root

The African American essayist, playwright, and novelist James Baldwin once said, *"Not everything that is faced can be changed, but nothing can be changed until it is faced."* How does one know that they are affected by historical trauma and how do they find out? The textbook answer would be to get a screening or assessment from a mental health professional, to uncover information, such as one's histories of trauma and experience with trauma-related symptoms, family history, and presenting problem.

Racism, oppression, poverty, and generations of state and local laws that supported legal discrimination such as Jim Crow and Black Codes, in addition to egregious acts like, lynching and racial profiling, also contribute to the many challenges found in families. African American families are all too familiar with these challenges, as they've acculturated to Western society throughout history.

Research findings have revealed that African Americans are predisposed to heightened stress, as a result of historical traumas they have experienced, and that actual (or perceived) racial discrimination has been found to negatively affect mental and physical health. In times of distress, the idea that one's present experience is due to unhealed childhood wounds may not be so obvious; therefore, seeking therapy to gain better insight may prove to be beneficial.

My therapeutic experience taught me that a family entrenched in their family history and culture has a better understanding of *how* and *why* they perceive the world around them as they do. In spite of these adversities, multiple aspects of family life have been found to be strengths, benefits, and protective factors in family life. One such strength is the ability to be resilient.

Through resilience and the connection created with extended family, these families survive. Also, feeling as though one is part of a community that holds traditions, religion, family structure, and organization in high regard, can help to solve challenges as they arise within a family.

Nevertheless, regardless of our strengths and innate survival instinct, as a culture, we have not been taught the importance of healing. Are our identities so deeply rooted in trauma that we are afraid to discover who we are outside of it?

Other than possible economic implications and other demographic barriers, one's beliefs and value systems may keep them away from seeking therapy.

There may be a stigma attached to therapy, consciously or subconsciously, that fuels the decision on whether or not to partake in therapy or therapeutic practices. This stigma may be associated with shame, embarrassment, or overall lack of trust. Fortunately, a professional therapeutic setting isn't the only option one has in seeking help or in-depth understanding of one's thoughts, feelings, and beliefs guide their behaviors and how to release the pain of historical trauma in healthy ways.

Heal De Tree

Throughout my youth, my village consisted of my family and friends, my James Island community, and my First Baptist Church home. As an adult, my village has expanded to include spiritual, mental, and physical health counselors and coaches, coworkers, and mentors.

Start where you are. Adopt the concept of beginning with the end in mind. When seeking a mental health provider, make certain that the mental health professional is competent in helping individuals or families cope and transition smoothly with the problems and challenges they face.

It is imperative that the therapist meets the individual or family where they are regarding their belief systems, organizational patterns, communications, and problem-solving abilities. With this knowledge, one can continue building on what works, and expel ideas in these areas that are not working, to allow a shift from one phase to another, while adapting to any change that may occur within the stages.

Moreover, a therapist decides if they are competent to treat a client, by not only the knowledge and skills acquired through their area of specialization but also through their knowledge of a client's culture. Cultural competency refers to knowledge, training, and life experiences acquired about a particular culture and includes being aware of one's values, culture, and biases.

To that end, it is crucial that the chosen professional is well-versed in the African American culture.

Therapists often use systematic principles, based on scientific methods, as a guiding framework for approaching issues a family or couple may bring to therapy, in an effort to make research-based clinical decisions. Treatment planning is centered on the development of a collaborative relationship that inspires hope and optimism, listens for strengths, and uses the beginner's mind.

On the other hand, when choosing not to participate in a clinical setting, or using alternative means of healing, self-help options rooted in data from existing research to help answer questions, solve or manage issues, is an alternative.

> *"You can accept or reject the way you are treated by other people, but until you heal the wounds of your past, you will continue to bleed. You can bandage the bleeding with food, with alcohol, with drugs, with work, with cigarettes, with sex, but eventually, it will all ooze through and stain your life. You must find the strength to open the wounds, stick your hands inside, pull out the core of the pain that is holding you in your past, the memories, and make peace with them."*
>
> -Iyanla Vanzant

Today, technology has made self-help books, articles, websites, and programs readily available and easily assessable to the general public. I am on a lifelong journey to discovering who I am, outside of the world telling me who I should be, with the intent of helping those along the way.

In my pursuit, I discovered *Post Traumatic Slave Syndrome* by Dr. Joy Degruy and *Black Rage* by Dr. William H. Grier and Dr. Price M. Cobs. These books gave me the "Aha" moments I needed for confirmation about what I learned through therapy and my studies. I have come to the conclusion that historical trauma can affect present-day experiences, leading to a multitude of adverse behaviors or historical trauma response features, resembling low self-esteem, dissociation, anger, hypervigilance, self-destructive behavior, and victim identity, to name a few.

This topic demands more attention, and I intend to do just that. We must all take an active role in the healing process of ourselves, our communities, our people, and our culture.

Black therapists are needed at the front lines to combat the war within, but you must first be willing to operate from a sense of self, and *tek cyear a de root.*

WHAT'S EATING YOU?
By Renetta D. Weaver, LCSW

4:34 a.m.

My Facebook Video Message:

"OMG, I can't believe today is the day. Today is Thursday, June the 16, 2016, and I'm here at Washington Hospital Center, about to go in and change my life (lets out breath) for the better (pause).

Today is the day that I'm having my procedure, Gastric Sleeve Surgery, and I'm so excited about it. This morning when I got on the scale, I was 235.7, and I started out (pause) ugh, my highest weight was 256.4, and I started out at 248.8, and I'm so excited about six months from now what things are going to look like. But umm... today is the day. I have a few butterflies; umm, that's just nervous excitement.

I can't believe that this is finally happening; this is such a gift to me. I really want to thank my friend for telling me about the surgery. I don't want to call her out because that's her personal business, but my friend basically had the surgery. She told me about it and gave me her surgeon's name and number.

So, umm, now it's my turn, and it's about 4:34 a.m. and I will have to check in at 5:30. My surgery starts at 7:30 a.m., and I should go in recovery about 9:30, so uhhh... I will be back and let you know how everything went. But just wanted to make this last recording before I go in and change my life.

And I thank God for this. I give God all the glory, honor, and praise and I pray that His hands will be with me and the surgery team and everybody that interacts with me this morning."

On June 16, 2016, I underwent Bariatric Surgery, commonly known as Weight Loss Surgery, and my procedure was the Vertical Sleeve Gastronomy. A year earlier, I had gotten up to my highest weight of 256.4, and I was wearing a size 3X top and a size 22 bottom on my 5'3 frame.

During the previous year, I had also gone to the Podiatrist to find out why it hurt to walk. I mean, I knew that I had flat feet, but I had stopped wearing high heels a long time ago, so I was wondering what was going on. That year, I was concerned about other health problems as well. For instance, every time I went to the doctor, I was informed that my blood pressure was extremely high. I would see the look of horror on the medical professional's face as they read the results on the machine, always getting asked about my drinking and smoking habits, of which I proudly denied both; however, they never asked about my eating... or *what was eating me!*

Ultimately, I made an appointment with a new doctor my husband had recommended. She was young, petite, and looked like she never had a weight problem in her life. I remember her handing me a list of dos and don'ts eat foods, while she tossed her hair, pranced around the office, and urged me to lose weight.

"So, how did it go?" asked my husband. With tears of frustration, I said, "I'm not ever going back to see that skinny bitch again. She doesn't know anything about what it's like to be overweight." I was so angry that she didn't understand that at my age and weight, as well as being an educated professional in the medical field, I already knew what and *what not* to eat at this stage of the game.

I had been on every diet known to man!

What I needed her to ask me was, *"What's Eating You?"*

The following year, I was assigned to a new doctor. I was so excited because I was hoping that this doctor would better understand my needs. He seemed to be seriously concerned about my high blood pressure and placed me on a water pill, HZTZ; the same medication that my mother had been prescribed. However, my mom has always been in great health and didn't need to start taking any medication until she was in her 70s. On the other hand, I was only in my early 40s when I needed to start taking it. I digress, anyway, as with any new medication, my doctor wanted me to come back in six months for a follow-up. He would always express concern that I hadn't lost any weight.

In fact, my weight was trending up.

Therefore, he recommended that I start going to the gym three times a week, for thirty minutes. Again, I was internally frustrated because here was another doctor that didn't seem to think that I knew what to do and had already attempted it.

Well, at the next follow-up appointment with my Primary Care Physician, my blood pressure concerned him so much that he placed me on a stronger blood pressure medication. I was no longer just taking the water pill, and whatever was in that new medication made me develop a persistent dry cough, and I noticed that my hair immediately thinned out, became dry and brittle, and begun falling out; resulting in two bald spots on the front and side of my scalp. I always had hang-ups about my hair, felt it wasn't good enough, and now I was losing it.

Another thing that concerned me was being told by my Primary Care Physician that I was pre-diabetic and that if I didn't change my diet and lose some weight, I was going to be placed on stronger maintenance medication.

At the same time, I had developed a severe case of dry and itchy skin, which first started on my arms and legs, and then subsequently spread all over my body.

No amount of scratching was enough to quell the itch, and sometimes, the vigorous scratching would wake my husband or cause blood to discharge from my broken skin. My doctor told me to change my washing powder, body soap, and body lotion. My husband bought me itch cream and ointment that only made me a white pasty mess.

Neither of those solutions were working.

I felt and knew that I had an internal itch that couldn't be satisfied by anything externally.

Again, I needed to be asked, *"What's Eating You?"*

After venting to my friend about my weight loss struggles, itchy skin, high blood pressure, and being pre-diabetic, she shared the benefits of weight loss surgery with me and gave me the number to the Bariatric Clinic, as well as the website. I didn't call right away, but I did my research and thought about it for a couple of months.

Another friend shared with me that her family member didn't have a good outcome when she underwent the Gastric Bypass because she ultimately ended up gaining all her weight back. Nevertheless, I was a daily witness of two of my friends who were rapidly losing inches and doing well after having the surgery.

So, right before Thanksgiving, 2015, I decided to call the Bariatric Office and schedule myself for the information seminar. I took my husband to the information seminar and finally felt like I found the place that understood my needs.

After years of feeling like I had lost control of my body, and that I was on a slow path to death, I now had hope. As my husband and I were leaving, I looked into his eyes and said, "I am having this surgery, and you can leave me if you want to." He responded, "I support you; do what you need to do."

Fast forward to April 5, 2016; it was my birthday dinner when I was surrounded by my family. I said, "I have an announcement, and no, I'm not pregnant." One of them asked, "What's the announcement?" I answered, "I am having Weight Loss Surgery in June." Immediately, everyone started questioning my decision; advising me on how I could just eat properly and exercise to lose weight. Then my brother asked my husband, "What do you think about this? Are you going to let her do this?"

My husband answered, "I can't stop her. Once she makes up her mind to do something, she's going to do it."

It was at that point that I said to my family, "I'm not asking for your permission, I'm just telling you, and you can be there or not be there. This time, I wrote my own permission slip." I informed them, "I'm tired of living my life to please other people, and I am the only one who knows what it feels like to live inside my body."

So, what did it feel like, you ask? Well, let me try to explain it to you. I did not commit any crime, but I judged myself guilty. I sentenced myself to a prison of pain, and became institutionalized, as I did over a 30-year bid.

Even with good behavior, my incarceration was marred with so many failed attempts to escape that I ended up spending most of it in solitary confinement.

My name is Renetta, and I want to share with you my story about living in a mental and emotional prison of pain. Inmate number 04051971, charged with being a victim of sexual assault by molestation, handcuffed in guilt and shame, clothed in obesity and placed in solitary confinement due to repeated problems with intimacy among the general population.

I was falsely accused of an act that was perpetrated by a fraud, a true deceiver, who made me a believer that I was all the negative adjectives such as ugly, bad, dirty, different, and unlovable. Most damaging was the feeling of being unworthy.

My experience of childhood sexual abuse and trauma at the tender age of eight produced in me a false belief of unworthiness that instantly turned into the mental bondage of self-limiting beliefs. I began to serve out my sentence, and as time passed over the years, I started believing that there was no way of escape from the captivity of the negative and painful emotions that I merely existed in.

For at least three decades, following the sexual abuse, I lived in a cell that weighed approximately three pounds and was about fifteen centimeters long; the average size of the human brain.

The size of my cell might sound small in weight and diameter, but that prison of pain was as large as a smoldering volcano that would often erupt in acts of self-destructive behavior and bouts of rage. For years, I was unable to walk in my purpose and live out my goals and dreams because my legs were shackled with self-hate. That self-hate was cemented with internalized depression along with externalized irritability, anger, and rage toward others.

My numerous attempts to break loose from that mental and emotional bondage failed miserably, and I was miserable. Each time I tried to escape, I found myself submerging deeper and deeper into the abyss of hopelessness and ultimately drowning in suicidal thoughts.

I did not want to die, but I did not know how else to escape from the pain of feeling dead inside. Even though I didn't have an actual attempt or plan, the self-neglect upon my body through un-protected sex and eating were acts of slow suicide. Considering how overwhelmed I was, mentally and emotionally, I can honestly say at that time in my life I would not have been mad if I did not wake up the next morning.

In my futile effort to numb myself from the pain of my scars, I used food as gauze to cover up my aching wounds that were ooz-ing with silent tears. These were the same tears that woke me up every morning at 3 a.m. as I muffled screams into my soaked pillow. I continued to float in the ocean of negative emotions; riding the waves of low self-esteem every time the tide of rejection by others rolled in.

I entered into relationships with cellmates who were also unable to escape from their mental incarceration.

Despite my feelings of inadequacy, I thought I could love them into freedom and unconsciously believed that my ability to do that would restore my worth and value. Although every relationship ended the same, I had a hard time admitting and accepting that my love was not enough to free them from their pain. Whenever they discovered that drinking and drugging weren't enough for them to break free from their prison of mental and emotional pain, my body became the wall that they punched, kicked, shoved, and sexed in their attempts to escape.

This cycle of physical abuse continued for years and fed into my belief system that I was not good enough and that my shortcomings caused someone to react in a hurtful and harmful way towards me. I thought I deserved it, feeling that I was to blame; I lost my confidence, my voice, walked on eggshells, became a people pleaser, and found myself in codependent relationships.

After years of attempting self-help, one day, I decided to get help. Through getting help, I learned that I wasn't responsible for the experience that happened to me, but I was responsible for how I would continue to experience life. That moment was a definite plot twist. I started to believe that someone out there had the keys to help me lose my mind from bondage so that I wouldn't lose my mind. I began to get honest with myself and finally admitted that I had problems and pain that I couldn't fix on my own.

I realized that my best thinking was like an outdated GPS which was stored with faulty pre-adolescent maps that navigated me in so many wrong directions.

Trying to escape on my own, I went as far as I could go until I found myself running on empty fumes and my life almost reached a dead end.

My ego was finally ready to admit that I need help!

DIFFERENT:
"Partly or totally unlike in nature, form, or quality."
-Merriam-Webster Dictionary

Different! Yeah, that's exactly how I felt after that; after being told by my mom that I was adopted. I remember crying and running out of the house into our brown family station wagon that was parked in our driveway. After that day, I started to act out and misbehave until my mother got fed up and said, "Look, I am your mother, and you are no different than your brothers, and I will spank you like I spank them."

Although hearing that made me feel good, I still felt different, and my self-view was forever changed. I started to notice that my looks were different; my dad and brothers were a beautiful dark complexion and my mother was a beautiful golden-brown complexion with long, soft, Indian hair and a curvy figure. Who was I?

Well, I felt like a jigsaw puzzle, and none of my family pieces fit. As a young child, feeling different is a contributing risk factor for vulnerability.

When I was a young girl, my family lived in the middle-class suburb area of Prince George's County called Clinton, MD. I loved growing up in Clinton, and I still have fond memories of how my friends and I used to walk and ride our bicycles miles away from home to visit each other. Like many of you reading this, I just had to be home by the time the street lights came on. Back then, it was even safe for my friends and me to play in the woods and tobacco fields, and we used those two as pathways to visit each other's neighborhoods.

I still remember, as clear as yesterday, when it stopped feeling so safe for me. It was a typical sunny and warm summer day when one of my friends, who lived two neighborhoods over, had navigated from her home, through the woods, and over to my house to play. My brothers who were in charge of babysitting me were in the house; down in the basement, listening to music on their 8-track tape player, smoking marijuana from a red bong, and having fun with their friends.

Me? Well, I was outside playing on the Sit and Spin. That's when Purple Lip Johnny appeared in my driveway, and at that moment, I still felt safe. You see, I had no reason not to feel safe around Purple Lip Johnny. He lived on the same street, and although it was up the street, his house was two doors away from my childhood babysitter's.

He also was very close friends with my brothers, so he was always at our house, and called my mother "mom."

Therefore, although my brothers and their friends were downstairs, it did not alarm me that Purple Lip Johnny would meet me upstairs in the foyer, while I was playing by myself. Unbeknownst to me, he had begun to groom me by showing me attention. Initially, I didn't think anything was weird about his attention towards me. However, I recollect the day he said to me, "You're so mature for your age."

As an eight-year-old, I was unsure of what that meant, but it made me feel weird inside.

My next memory was of me standing with him in my dark bathroom shower, as he had his hands under my blue turtleneck shirt, with his fingertips touching and rubbing me. I honestly don't know how I ended up there, or what happened after, but I do recall knowing that I did not enjoy it, yet I was afraid to tell anyone.

Well, back to that day when I was playing in my driveway with my childhood friend, Purple Lip Johnny walked over to us and asked, "Y'all want to go have some fun?" My friend and I eagerly answered, "Yes!" He then invited us to come with him up the street to his house. Now, I had never been to his house, but I really didn't have a reason to say 'no' because he was a neighbor; who was like a brother, who was always at my house, and who told us we were going to have fun. And, of course, my eight-year-old brain wanted to have fun.

Off to Purple Lip Johnny's house, we went.

I can see my younger *self* walking up the driveway into the carport area where the side door to his house was located.

My friend and I entered his home and were escorted through the fully furnished dining room, through the kitchen, and down the dark hallway towards the bedrooms. He sent my friend into one bedroom and took me with him into his parent's bedroom.

I recall the dimly sunlit room was tightly furnished with a multi-drawer brown oak dresser topped with a large mirror, a brown oak chest of drawers, a very large unmade bed with beige colored sheets, perfumed with the stale smell of cigarettes and beer in the air. After standing for a few seconds, he instructed me to sit on the edge of the bed, told me to lie down, and then he removed my bottoms.

He then began trying to force his 18-year-old erect penis into my intact hymen, eight-year-old vagina. I can still feel the excruciating pain as he continued to forcefully attempt to penetrate me but couldn't.

He finally abandoned his efforts.

My relief was short lived as he summoned me over and I found myself standing in front of him as he leaned against the long oak dresser.

If I close my eyes, I can distinctly remember the smell of his penis as he placed it against my lips and forced it into my mouth. I obeyed him as he instructed me on how to perform oral sex on him. He told me to stop and invited my friend into the room. Once in the room, he told her that I had done a good job and now he wanted me to show her how to do it.

Just as Purple Lip Johnny was about to have me continue, we were interrupted by the noise of the house side door opening. Instantly, Purple Lip Johnny ushered my friend and me into the shower of his parent's bathroom. We stayed there while we heard his father's loud footsteps move throughout the house. I guess his father was only coming home for lunch because he soon left back out. That is when Purple Lip Johnny escorted us out of the shower, through the bedroom, back down the dark hallway, back through the kitchen, to the living room... and just before we exited through the side door, he warned us not to tell anyone what happened, or we would be in big trouble.

After we agreed, he told us to run down the backside of his house, and down the hill through a neighbor's yard to another area of my neighborhood; all designed to conceal that I was ever at his home.

Once we got down the hill, my friend left through the woods and I went home. She and I have never talked to one another about this, even though we attended elementary, middle, and high school together, have both seen and talked to each other following graduation, and are active Facebook friends to this day.

Looking back on my story of trauma in the form of childhood sexual abuse, I now realize that this is where I had stopped breathing, and my heart had stopped beating. It was as if I had taken in a deep breath of what all five of my senses felt at that moment. I can still visualize his house and his father's room; I can still feel the uncomfortable touch of his hands; I can still taste his penis in my mouth; I can still smell the stale cigarettes and beer, and I can still hear him warn me, "You better not tell anybody."

When trauma occurs to a child or young adult, he or she gets stuck in their psychological and emotional development. My child abuse history dates back to my primary years, and that is where my emotional *self* had been trapped for years. I was indeed very sad, lonely, and depressed as a young girl and no one seemed to notice because no one said anything to me; not even when I cried every day in my classroom. But it was hard for my mom not to notice because I was irritable and angry towards her all the time. I could not understand why my mother was not there to protect me, why she continued to allow my abuser back into our home, and why she continued to allow him to call her 'mom.'

My expression of anger towards my mother was also there because my childhood emotional brain blamed her for not knowing something I thought she should have known. My feelings towards my mom were also because she never talked to me about sex. Her way of talking to me about sex was to give me five books called the "Life Cycle."

They were informative books about everything from necking and petting, all the way to sexual intercourse. However, if I had a question about any of it, I knew I could not ask her.

While my mother didn't educate me about sex, she sure did scold me when she found my diary which made any content in a Zane novel read like a children's book. The pages of my diary were filled with graphic details of how I engaged in, and enjoyed, having sex when I was the tender age of fifteen.

One line I will never forget is when I said, "He fucked me so good from the back that I was blind."

Yes, I think we were both horrified when she read that.

She told my dad, and he said, "Look, if you are going to do stuff like that, don't write it down." I was humiliated that my parents learned about my dirty little secret. Once again, the natural, pleasurable act of sex was turned into something that made me view myself as disgusting. Thus, along with becoming sexualized, I developed a lot of guilt and shame around my body and the act of sex. However, my feelings of guilt and shame didn't stop my body from enjoying the benefits of sex; the orgasms, the attention, the acceptance, and the ability to please and get what felt like love.

The experience of sexual abuse taught me that sex is what a male wanted, and the more I learned to be good at it, the more loveable and wanted I would become. Therefore, as a teenager, I began to use sex as a tool to get love and acceptance; although it was temporary because it was always gone once the sex was over.

Sex became like a drug, and I would get a rush every time I engaged in the act. Then, the high would be gone when the guy was gone, and my mood went from elevated to deflated.

From youth into adulthood, I was extremely depressed, and I beat myself up with the gloves of internal anger. I had a lot of reasons to be angry, and other than expressing it towards my mom, who was safe because she had to love me, I couldn't bring myself to express it towards Purple Lip Johnny. Every time he came around me, my insides wanted to scream, but the only thing that came from my mouth was a smile.

At an early age, I learned to wear the mask of happiness to cover up my true feelings of sadness in public. This set me up for years of having poor boundaries and being a doormat.

However, in private with my family, I displayed all the symptoms of depression and indicators that something was wrong, such as excessive sleeping and crying, that used to frustrate my mother to no ends because she didn't know how to fix what was wrong. I desperately wanted to be able to talk to my mom about what I was going through, but I just didn't know how.

As a result, I continued to internalize my pain and spent many years stuck in a cycle of what initially felt like acceptance, yet always ended in rejection. It seemed that no matter how good I put it down in the bedroom, it never proved good enough to get a guy to choose me as his mate.

What I wanted and needed more than anything was to be chosen. Instead, I would always find myself stuck in the friend zone; friends with benefits, of course.

This experience of repeated rejection placed layers on the foundation toward my feeling unworthy, undesirable, and unlovable. Day in and day out, I cried so much that my eyes would always be puffy and swollen shut in the morning. Not knowing any other way to help me, my mother would give me eye gel to help me further disguise my pain.

In her efforts to cheer me up, my mother used to say to me that life is what you make it, so I tried hard to pull myself out of those feelings of depression by reading the Bible and crying out to God in prayer, but I was stuck in unbearable pain. And my prayers went from *Lord, please take away my pain* to *Lord, please take away my life.*

I had gone from being sad to suicidal, and the only thing that kept me from swallowing the bottle of pills in our medicine cabinet was that I was not courageous enough. But, I can honestly say that I was praying for God not to wake me up in the morning. To escape these feelings, I turned to food as another source of escape and pleasure.

Recently, sorting through some childhood photos, I noticed the obvious difference in my physique from age eight to age ten. If the body keeps the score, my body was losing a wrestling match against life; being pinned under the weight of trauma symptoms.

Not only was I feeling the mental and emotional weight of my secret sexual shame, but I was also feeling the weight of keeping other family secrets like my parents fighting about my older brothers' alcohol and marijuana use. My mother's attempt to rescue and protect my brothers was not enough to keep my dad from putting them out of the house.

They were my best friends and used to play games with me like swinging me in a blanket and making me a human cannonball by kicking me off their feet. They were also my babysitters who let me sit in the tall chair and wash the dishes when my parents weren't home, and we were road dogs. They took me everywhere with them, and when they left home, I became extremely lonely. They were my first teachers of what relationships with men looked like, which was abandonment!

After my brothers left, a summer visit from one of my favorite cousins brought much joy to our home. I remember standing in our kitchen with my cousin, and I am not sure what I was eating, but I remember her saying, "You better be careful; you are going to get fat." I said to her, "I don't care because food is good." My childhood brain learned to associate food with pleasure.

Consequently, whenever I felt sadness, rejection, loneliness, or some other feeling of pain and discomfort, I turned to food for relief. Just like any drug of choice, food gave me an escape, and as time passed, I needed to consume more and more food to fill that empty space. I swallowed many thoughts and stuffed down an enormous amount of feelings that my body could no longer hide.

My outer appearance began to reflect my internal experience, and the heaviness of carrying so many secrets added up to extra inches and increased pounds on the scale. This extra weight contributed to the negative body image issues I had first developed from the sexual trauma. Now, my body, the only thing I felt was desirable *about* me, was no longer desirable *to* me.

Being overweight remarkably impacted my self-esteem; causing me to develop many self-limiting beliefs. I never thought I was good enough, so I stopped doing things that would cause me to be seen.

I attempted to engage in psychotherapy twice before, but I wanted my mom to come, and since she refused, I stopped going. This time, I decided to go just for me; putting all of my cards on the table and allowing myself to explore and examine a range of difficult thoughts, memories, and behaviors.

During my Psychological Evaluation, I was a little afraid that I wouldn't be a candidate for weight loss surgery due to sharing my story and expressing my emotions, but I did it anyway. I couldn't help but think about how vulnerable my therapy clients must feel when they worry about the consequences of getting honest. At that very moment, I was so grateful for that environment of confidentiality and non-judgmental positive regard.

Thankfully, the Psychologist told me that he thought that I was a good candidate for surgery and that losing the weight would be healing for me. He did warn me that I would need to find another way to deal with my emotions, other than eating.

I took heed to his words because that is the same thing that I convey to the group members at my addictions treatment facility. If nothing changes, nothing changes!

An honest program of recovery requires you to change people, places, and things. Currently, I am two years post-surgery, and I am down to a size 12 and weigh 180, but I realize that my doctor didn't do surgery on my brain.

I'm finally ready to address the root of my problems, and I'm walking the talk by re-engaging in psychotherapy.

I've been told that my story is too heavy. My response is, "If it's too heavy for you to read, imagine what it felt like for me to carry it for all these years."

In sharing my story with you, I have become fully aware of the internal weight of silencing my voice and holding in mental and emotional pain.

For years, I thought I was covering up with a fake smile, but my emotions started showing up as excess body weight. I truly want to share my story for anyone out there that has a similar story, those who have borne the burdens of surviving trauma and have felt the heaviness of carrying their mental, emotional and physical weight.

Now, I have just one question:

"What's Eating You?"

I DON'T BELIEVE IN MONSTERS

By A.C. Fowlkes, PhD

I was raised in a hyper-religious household. I struggle to characterize it this way because I don't want to be unfair in my representation of our home; however, I really don't know what else to call it. I have witnessed more than my fair share of exorcisms, anointing oil, screams of "Come out in the name of Jesus!", people vomiting and coughing, crying and wailing, passing gas and belching, slobbering and snotting.

That's how the demons come out. They come out in bodily secretions. They come out in tears and vomit. They come out in flatulence. And you must be very, very careful because they come out seeking another host. They look to enter into whoever is not spiritually strong enough to resist them.

Children are easy targets. Sometimes they would usher us to the back of the church, "Somebody get the kids... move them back. They're too close." We would huddle in the back of the church; staring in terror. If we had been in a large building, ushering us away would have made more sense, but we weren't. It was impossible to stay in the sanctuary and be more than thirty feet away from the possessed man or woman who was actively shrieking and vomiting.

I knew from an early age that frogs represented demons. You should never touch them. I mean never; not even the fake ones because frog statues also represent demons.

I made eye contact with an owl once. I was standing outside one night, and an owl was perched on a power line. He kept his body still and turned his head in that way only owls can. He turned his head and stared at me. We stared at each other.

And then, I remember getting home later that night and saying, *"An owl stared at me tonight while I was outside. We just sat there and stared at each other for a while."* The response was swift and deliberate, "Owls represent demons." I recoiled for a brief second, and then in a moment of pride, I said, *"Well, I stared right at him, and I wasn't afraid of him,"* a hint of a smile across my face. My mother looked at me and said, "It doesn't matter that you weren't afraid of him. The real question is... why wasn't he afraid of you?"

I was in church almost every day of the week. Monday was Bible College. Tuesday was intercessory prayer. Wednesday was Bible study. I don't recall what Thursday was, but Friday was "Teen Night." Saturdays were hit and miss, but I remember many a Saturday going to the church to clean or pray or otherwise get the "house in order."

And Sunday? Well, on Sundays, we were in church from 9:00 a.m. until about 3:00 p.m., although some Sundays we didn't get out of church until 6:00 or 7:00 p.m.

My life pretty much revolved around spiritual practice, and by the time I was in middle school, I was seeing angels and demons. I'm not sure what most middle schoolers did when they weren't in school, but I spent a great deal of my time in worship. I remember playing worship songs on repeat in the living room and dancing before God. This was one of my favorite pastimes, something I did when I was home alone.

The first time I saw angels I was doing just that. There was a song on repeat—a song of repentance, a song of worship—and I was dancing before the Lord. I can still hear the song lyrics clearly:

"You're calling my name to come into your arms, to be safe from fear and harm. Knowing this but I still choose to go my way. And you still say. You say that I am He, who will supply your every need. Oh Lord, I've sinned, but you're still calling my name."[2]

The song played over and over, and I danced and danced. And then it happened. My eyes were closed. I heard a voice just as clear as the voice in your head right now reading the words off of this page. He told me I was safe, that angels were surrounding me to protect me. And then there was a nudge, not a physical nudge but a spiritual one, something within me that told me to open my eyes.

When I opened my eyes, I saw angels around me in a massive circle, and they were wearing the whitest white I had ever seen. Their wings were extended, and they were positioned in such a way that each one's wings overlapped with the wings of the angel on either side. I remember marveling at the sight. I slowly turned around, a complete 360-degree circle, and I saw that they encompassed me completely.

---

[2] *"Calling My Name;* Hezekiah Walker, Family Affair 2: Live At Radio City Music Hall, 2002

I heard his voice again. He told me why their wings were over-lapping. He explained that their wings' overlapping ensured that there was no point of entry. I was safe. I stood there, slowly spin-ning, mouth agape in astonishment and then I did it; I did what we all do.

I blinked. And when I opened my eyes, they were gone.

Seeing angels never bothered me. My angels were warm and inviting. They made me feel safe. In order to get to me, you would have to get past my angels. And I had a lot of them! The demons, though... the demons were much less fun. I began to see them at school. I would see them attached to people, literally attached to their backs and I could see the vice that they represented.

For each person it was different.

Lunchtime was particularly bad; I would walk into the cafeteria and be overwhelmed. There were so many kids in there at one time. And there were so many demons. They were everywhere, attached to the backs of, not all, but many of the students. You see, there is a difference between possession and oppression. Demons did not possess my friends but oppressed them. The demons had not made their way inside of them, but they had attached them-selves to them and were impacting them despite not having fully taken possession of them.

As you can imagine, simply sitting down at the table next to a person with a demon on their back was not an option. Demons are always looking for a new host, remember? So, I prayed in tongues under my breath, and I paced. I got in and out of the cafeteria as quickly as I could, and once I was outside, I went through a ritual of binding, loosing, casting down, and rendering inoperable, to make sure that I too was not possessed or oppressed by the demons in the cafeteria. Later, I shared my experiences with the members of my church. They said that I was "seeing in the realm of the spirit."

I don't know if that was a true description of what was occurring in my 8th-grade brain, but what I do know is that I hated going in the cafeteria.

It was in the sixth grade when I realized that I was attracted to girls. My very first crush was on a girl named Jenna. Her father and my mother worked together. She was beautiful. She had long blonde hair that reached her waist.

She was popular. I wasn't.

My first kiss took place in the sixth grade. It wasn't Jenna. It was instead the girl who lived across the street. She moved to my neighborhood, and we became fast friends. She liked to eat carrots, a lot. I'd never been a fan of carrots, but after a while, they began to grow on me. One day she was at my house, and we were hanging out in my room and, to be honest, I can't even tell you what happened. All I know is we kissed. There were no tongues involved. She lay on top of me and pressed her body against mine, and we kissed for what seemed like an eternity. Our lips were pressed tightly closed, but we moved our heads back and forth as if they weren't. I remember going to my mother after this happened.

I remember saying, "Mom, I think I'm gay!"

Her response, "Why do you say that?"

I answered, "Because the girl across the street and I kissed, and I don't know what I felt, but I felt it!"

My mother shrugged it off and said that we were simply exploring our bodies. That was a good enough explanation for me. I went on later that year to date a couple of boys in the neighborhood. We never kissed, and I never felt for them what I had felt for Jenna or the girl across the street. I spent the next couple of years focusing on God and basketball.

Everything was okay for the time being (well, as it relates to my sexual orientation) until I reached the 8th grade.

My world came crumbling down on me in the 8th grade. I was beginning to notice girls even more, and I would find myself drawn to them in a way that I didn't seem to be drawn to boys. I remember it like it was yesterday. I went to my mother, and I told her I needed to speak to her. She was sitting on the balcony of our apartment. She sat in a chair, and I sat on the ground beside her.

I was crying. I was afraid. I was in distress.

I sat there with my mother, and I spoke to her through my tears, "Mom, I think I am gay."

Her response was the same as it was two years earlier, "Why do you say that?"

I said, "Because I'm noticing girls in a way that I'm not noticing boys. And I feel uncomfortable in the locker room because there are all of these girls getting undressed, and I feel like I am looking at them in a way that I shouldn't."

My mother's response this time was much different than the response from a couple of years ago. She said, "The devil's trying to get you."

I cried harder.

It was around this same period in my life that I saw the demon of homosexuality cast out of someone for the first time. I had always been taught that homosexuality was a sin. Sometimes homosexuality was referred to as a demon, and other times it was referred to as an unclean spirit, but it was always referred to as evil.

I was in the 8th grade and struggling with same-sex attraction the first time I saw the demon of homosexuality cast out of someone. I knew her personally, and I knew her well. She was a member of our church, and she had a budding musical career. She had been gone for a while touring, and when she returned the spirit of homosexuality had attached itself to her.

I will never forget seeing her surrounded by the church leaders. They were speaking in tongues fervently, and when they weren't speaking in tongues, they were binding and loosing. They were decreeing and declaring. They were commanding and taking dominion over. They were casting back to the pits of hell and rendering inoperable.

She was surrounded by them. She was on her knees, bent over in what appeared to be immense anguish. She was vomiting and sobbing. Mucus ran from her nose, tangling with lines of thick saliva as she heaved. This was one of those times that they ushered us to the back of the sanctuary.

She began to cough and belch. The demons were coming out. They had us go into the hallway this time. The back of the sanctuary wasn't far enough, not for this demon—not for a demon as dangerous as homosexuality. "Get the children out of here! Get the children out! Go! Go! Go!"

I suppose the exorcism was successful. We never talked about it after that. She went on the road again. When she returned, she was found to be unclean. The church leaders surrounded her yet again. She collapsed to the floor on her knees and began to vomit as they cast out the demon of homosexuality in the name of Jesus!

And thus, the cycle began.

Every time she went on the road, she would become possessed or oppressed by the demon of homosexuality, and every time she returned they would usher us to the back of the church (sometimes even into the hallway) to protect us as they exorcised her demons. I think of how much the situation impacted me, and I feel a sense of sadness for her younger sister. She had a sister who was near my age. The whole situation terrified her. She used to sleep at night with a Bible on her chest. It made complete sense to do so.

After all, her older sister was possessed.

I spent the next several years trying not to be gay. I begged God to remove the unclean desires from me. I prayed, and I cried. I prayed, and I cried. I fasted, and I prayed, and I cried. I turned over my plate, I fasted, and I prayed, and I cried. I lay prostrate before the Lord, and I begged. I fasted and prayed and cried and begged.

No matter how much I cried out before God, I could not seem to get un-gay. I was afraid of eternal damnation. You know, *the wages of sin is death* (Romans 6:23). Even if I didn't act on it, I was having unclean thoughts about women, and the Good Book says, *as a man thinketh in his heart so is he* (Proverbs 23:7). So, even though I wasn't acting on it, and I was begging God to remove the taste from my lips because I could not tame my affection for the same sex, I was doomed.

I spent the rest of my teenage years, begging God to make me un-gay. Nothing I did seemed to work. I turned over my plate, I fasted, I prayed, I cried, I begged, and I dated boys.

Still gay. I could not make it stop. Most painful was the assumption by those in the church that I must be gay as a result of not having enough faith to experience deliverance.

I was a failure.

All I needed was faith 'the size of a mustard seed,' and it was obvious I failed to have even that much. I was broken. I was confused. I was lost.

When I started college was when things began to shift. When people could no longer blame my attire on my being a tomboy the heat got turned up. I was oppressed by an unclean spirit, and I needed deliverance. I wasn't around the same church folks anymore, but it didn't matter.

Even though I was all the way across the country, I was surrounded by people that believed the same as my old church family had. And that's when it started... when they started calling me up to the altar for deliverance; when they started laying hands on me and casting out homosexuality.

I had become the person on their knees, doubled over in anguish, sobbing. Were the demons coming out through my tears? That's one of the ways demons come out, remember? I knelt there sobbing and heaving as they bound and loosed and cast out and cast down to the pits of hell and rendered inoperable.

I sobbed as they exorcised the demon of homosexuality.

When it was over, I continued to lay on the altar, physically exhausted, spiritually broken. I stood up slowly, the anointing oil still glimmering on my forehead. They told me they loved me and asked me to come back and fellowship with them next Sunday. I slowly walked out of the front doors of the church, touching my forehead and feeling the residue of the anointing oil. I had been delivered.

The demon was gone.

At just that moment, I lifted my head. The sun was beginning to set, and it was time to go home. I turned toward my car, and as

I did, a beautiful woman walked past me... I was attracted to her. I lowered my head in shame. I was exhausted. I was depleted. I was defeated.

I was gay.

There is something about being viewed as evil that is damaging to the psyche, particularly if that which makes you evil is something that is beyond your control. I was raised in an environment where homosexuality was believed to be the manifestation of a spirit of perversion. How does one reconcile oneself with that?

Perhaps if my attraction to women had actually been a "lifestyle choice" and I had simply purposed in my heart to live a life of sin, I would have been less affected emotionally by the prevailing opinion that I was somehow unclean.

But that was not my truth. I loved God with all my heart, and I didn't want to be like this. I didn't want to be gay. I was begging God to deliver me, to save my soul from eternal damnation. Despite my earnest pleas, I remained perverse.

God was refusing to deliver me.

Notice I say refusing. I never considered, even for a moment, that he was unable to deliver me. I hadn't been raised to believe that such a thing was possible.

God, as I knew him, was a God without limitation. So, I found myself in the unfortunate position of knowing in my heart that I had done all that I could do, to no avail. I had repented and placed it at his feet only to have him deny me. I was at the end of my rope. I did not know what else to do.

God's refusal to deliver me from the spirit of homosexuality represented, in my mind, the difference between life and death, the difference between Heaven and Hell, the difference between respite and torture.

And I mean this literally, not figuratively.

I truly believed that because I was gay, death, hell, and torture were my lot; not only in life, but also in death.

The depression I experienced was profound. Having others believe that I was an abomination was damaging, but far more damaging than that was the fact that I believed it myself. I had listened to my elders, and years of doing so had led to a profound self-hatred and internalized homophobia.

I wish I could say my situation was unique in some way, a fluke of some sort, but sadly, to say so would be dishonest. I have met countless individuals who were subjected to similar teachings. My experiences with the church were highly damaging, as were my experiences with well-meaning individuals whose teachings perpetuated my self-loathing.

I grew up to have my share of issues, but I am fortunate to be at a place in my journey where I have the courage and the resolution necessary to share my story with others.

Sadly, not everyone made it. Some have lost their lives at the hands of someone who hates them simply for existing. Others have lost their lives at their own hands.

Hatred (whether directed outward or inward) is a formidable foe that quickly siphons reason. I stand here today not because I am immune. In the past, I too have been concerned for my safety at the hands of people who despise me simply for existing. I have considered taking my own life when agonizing over my inability to change the orientation of my affections.

If I were to be completely honest with you, I think I am alive today, in part, because I walked away from the church in my early 20s. After years of begging God to set me free and trying to understand why he wouldn't, I walked away.

I couldn't reconcile myself with the notion of a just and loving God sentencing me to an eternity of torture and despair because of something I was *unable* to control, and he was *unwilling* to control. I could not in good faith continue to serve a God who was at worst sadistic and at best callous.

So... I walked away. I walked away from all of it. I walked away from the church. I walked away from God. And I truly believe it saved my life.

You may be readying yourself for an argument against the church. There is no need to, as I have no such argument to present; quite the contrary. In spite of my experiences (or perhaps because of my experiences), I am now a licensed minister. Still, you may be taken aback by the supernatural experiences that I recounted in the text (i.e., seeing angels and demons).

To be honest, I went through a period when it scared me. I have since accepted the fact that I am a seer.

This fact has been both confirmed and affirmed, and I am now an ordained prophet. You might assume, based on the stories I have shared about my upbringing, that I have a relationship with my mother that is strained or fraught with pain, distrust, and unresolved issues.

I don't.

To be clear, my mother is the strongest woman I know. To say I admire her is an understatement. She is my hero in many respects.

You see, this chapter is not about shortcomings; it is instead about the resilience of the human spirit. This chapter is about my journey from a place of self-loathing to a place of self-acceptance and love. This chapter is about how I went from seeing monsters everywhere (including within myself) to not believing in monsters at all.

I am a licensed clinical psychologist. I was drawn to mental health as a career field for various reasons. First and foremost, my mother is a therapist. I remember hearing her stories as a kid and being intrigued by her work. She would take me to her office when I was in elementary school. I would sit at her desk and color while she had therapeutic sessions elsewhere in the building. Now and then, I would hear her discuss a case. She never disclosed any information that would make the client identifiable.

I recognize this fact only in hindsight because, at the time, I had absolutely no interest in the identity of the person being discussed. I was more interested in the actions of her clients than their identity. I remember one day she and I discussed the topic of safety and whether her work had ever caused her to be concerned for her safety. She told me about a time when a client became infatuated with her and began stalking her. I remember her saying, "That's why I never drive straight home."

She went on to explain that she would drive around for a while to ensure that no one was following her before she came home to my sister and me.

Thinking on it now, I realize that my response to that story and others like it was less so one of fear and more so one of intrigue. I've always been drawn to psychopathology. I may not have officially taken an abnormal psychology class until I was in college, but I was well versed in the symptoms of common mental health diagnoses at a much younger age.

As a child I often found myself analyzing the behaviors of people and attempting to diagnose them. My interest in abnormal psychology was based on more than my mother's work. There was a lot of "abnormal" to be witnessed within my own family such as lengthy stays in mental institutions, the mysterious deaths of family pets, and that uncle everyone knew to never be alone with (to name a few).

There was a lot I didn't understand, and even more that I could not reconcile myself with; like, the suicide of my little brother, the fact that I was molested by a prominent member of my church, or the fact that I have been sexually assaulted (I use that word only because it is too painful to say raped) more times than I can recall.

I suppose all of these things worked in concert to push me toward mental health as a profession. And not only mental health, but I have spent more than half of my career working with a population that many refuse to work with; the pariah of our communities: sex offenders, and not just any sex offenders, but some of the most sexually deviant offenders in the country.

For example, I worked with a man once (we'll call him Stan) who was very sick. Stan had what we call zoophilia (you may know it as bestiality). When I started working with Stan, he had already had sexual contact with over 75 dogs and one dead deer. To make matters more disturbing, Stan had gone through the process of training his dogs to penetrate him anally. So, when I say he had sex with 75 dogs, what I am saying is he trained at least 75 dogs to mount him and have anal sex with him.

As I said, Stan was very sick. I have spent a significant portion of my career working with people like Stan.

I'll give you another example: let's call her Sarah. Sarah was a pedophile. She had victimized several small children, and she was very specific in her preferences. Sarah had "a type." In fact, she could tell you exactly what her "type" was. She preferred children four and under, who were of a fair complexion. She preferred they had curly hair and were bow-legged. She liked them to be old enough to walk (or waddle) but not old enough to be in school or communicate effectively.

Sarah was also very sick.

One of the perks of mental health is that you can choose the population you work with. I could have worked with any population, but I chose to work with them. And, more importantly, I was really good at it.

My patients often made significant progress. I didn't shame them or berate them. I extended compassion to them, but I also held them accountable. I aimed to truly understand them, and I challenged their cognitive distortions with laser-pointed focus. My coworkers and supervisors would often comment on the quality of the work I was doing with my clients and the gains they were making in treatment. I had patients asking if they could be on my caseload because they truly desired to change and had heard of my work.

I also had others who avoided me because they too had heard of my work and they weren't interested in changing.

Why this population? Why was I so good with this population? Of all the populations to choose from, why was I drawn to this one? That is a fair question, and I will try my best to answer it.

I'll say it like this: It is hardly a coincidence that I literally cannot tell you the number of times that I have been raped, but I became a certified sex offender treatment provider.

It is hardly a coincidence that I have a sense of compassion for this population and that I view them as chronically ill instead of as morally bankrupt.

See, the person who raped me was someone I loved deeply. He was someone who I desperately wanted to get help. He was someone I trusted. And while I cried myself to sleep many a night, I hoped that he would change at some point.

Rape is not always someone screaming and thrashing and fighting someone off them. Sometimes rape looks very different. Sometimes rape looks like having your clothes forcibly taken from you so that you are naked and unable to run for help, then being thrown onto a bed and having a phone book opened up and placed on top of you, while being repeatedly punched through the phone book so that you feel the impact of the blow, but there are no knuckle prints left behind. Then, after you have been beaten to the point of submission, having him get on top of you and have his way with you as you lie there, defeated and crying silently.

That is one of the rapes I actually remember.

I had been screaming for help through the entire beating, no one came to my aid (despite the fact that there was someone in the next room). I can't say I screamed "no" by the time he got on top of me. I had just taken a significant beating and didn't have it in me to scream, or even fight for that matter. So, I just lay there, defeated and motionless, and cried.

Our relationship was like many abusive relationships. When things were good, they were really good, and when things were bad, they were really bad. He almost killed me on more than one occasion. I remember saying to him that I was afraid he was going to kill me one day.

His reply, *"I would never kill you on purpose."*

Was he a monster? No. He had his own traumatic history. Nothing quite like the things he did to me, but trauma nonetheless. And hurt people, left to their own devices, often go on to hurt others. I think that was the case with him. Eventually, I left. It took multiple attempts (or should I say multiple restraining orders) and literally moving across the country, but I got away from him.

The impact that relationship had on me was lasting. It framed a lot of my experiences moving forward. In some ways, this proved to be unhealthy, and I mistreated the first couple of people I was with romantically after that relationship ended. But, in some ways, the impact it had on me was helpful. I think one of the ways it helped me most was that it gave me the ability to look at someone who does terrible things and not see a terrible person, but instead a person who does terrible things.

And that distinction, however slight, allowed me to look at people who had done the unthinkable and see them as they truly were—hurt, lost, misguided.

That is not to say people should not be held accountable. I am a firm believer in the experiencing of the natural consequences of your actions, be that incarceration, limitations on your freedom, mandated treatment, heightened monitoring in the community, etc. But, I believe just as strongly in redemption. I believe that even those who have committed terrible acts are deserving of compassion.

So, I coined the phrase "Compassionate Accountability," or "warm courage"; which perfectly sums up my treatment approach. It's not that I am saying that you are right. It's that even those who have done wrong deserve compassion.

As therapists, I think we can often identify moments in our development as clinicians that were transformative for us. The moments that helped us define who we were in this space. I'd like to share one of my stories with you.

I was facilitating a process group with female sex offenders. On this particular day, one of my clients was sharing a therapeutic homework assignment with the group so she could receive feedback from her peers and me. In the assignment, she had to answer some pointed questions about her offense and the underlying motivations of her behavior.

She became emotional while sharing the assignment.

After she finished reading her assignment to the group, she looked at me with a pained look on her face and said, "I feel like a monster. Am I a monster?"

She was looking at me, and it was clear to me that the words I said at that moment would shape her perspective of herself in a way that would not easily be undone. She looked at me with an aching in her eyes that is difficult to describe. She was waiting to see what I would say, waiting to see how I would define her in relationship to her past actions.

The other group members looked on as well.

It was clear she was not the only one on in the room with that question. She was just the only one brave enough to ask it. My co-facilitator looked on, wondering what I might say. And, in that instant, much more than a treatment modality was born; a worldview was born.

I looked directly into her eyes and said to her, with good conscience and clear mind, *"I don't believe in monsters."*

Relief washed over her. I was her treatment provider. I knew her deepest, darkest secrets, and as a result of that I was the voice she cherished more than any other at that juncture in her life. And I had affirmed her. I had given her permission to love herself. I had given her permission to begin the process of self-forgiveness. I had given her permission to start the process of healing. And I had done all of that with one simple yet weighted phrase, "I don't believe in monsters."

I've been asked how I could believe such a thing. I've come to realize over time that my beliefs are directly attributable to my past experiences, however difficult they might have been. It was my journey to self-love (despite the teachings of the church) that forged within me a steadfast belief that I am not a monster. And it was the repeated abuse at the hands of someone I loved that taught me others aren't monsters either.

We are all just people, trying to make sense of a very complicated world. I live my life by two very simple rules now: *Love God* and *Love people*.

The journey to get here was agonizing, but the result is one that I deeply cherish. And so, I leave you with this:

"I see you. I love you. I affirm you.
And never forget that you are worthy of redemption."

BLACK MINDS IN MEDITATION

By Daphne Fuller, LPC

Mornings were the worst for me. And, although I could escape my pain through sleep during the night, each morning, as the sun would peer through my curtains, my heart would fill with despair and a feeling of doom would overcome me.

I was sad, as I had found myself in a number of either mentally, emotionally, or physically abusive relationships throughout my life, to include the one I had with myself.

By age 20, I was a single mother in my second year of college, with a new baby boy. Daily, I was faced with the disappointing reality that I had to deal with this deep sadness in my heart once again, feeling alone, even though I had friends around me. I felt as if no one would understand.

My mother wanted more for me and instilled in me to respect myself, that boys meant me no good, and to make something of myself. You see she had lost both parents by the age of 18 and was a single mother to my older brother and later I was born. She had married my stepfather by the time I was four. My mom raised me in the church, doing everything she could to protect me from poor choices and people she believed would not be beneficial to me.

She just wanted me to enjoy life without worry, wanting better for me. I would say that growing up I was well taken care of, sheltered and often not allowed to hang out like my peers; plus living on the outskirts of town proved not to have much action!

Being sheltered made me curious as to what my mother was protecting me from because I would hear how much fun others my age were having; the things that they were able to do, and the places they were able to go. I wanted to be accepted, finding myself in a culture where sex and domestic violence was normal for young teens in relationships in my small town. I knew about other friends and teens in my town having sex, getting pregnant, having abortions, cheating, being cheated on, having low self-worth and being victims of domestic violence.

This was looked upon as normal, although my family life was not like this at all. That is just the way it was or how it felt for me. Maybe everyone wasn't doing it.

By the time I was 15, I had my first boyfriend, which turned out to be a physically and mentally abusive relationship. My grades were good, and I was involved in track, cross country, and basketball, going through life as if these things were fine. However, I can remember having my clothes and shoes taken by him, and being punched in the eye, leaving a mark, for no reason at all, other than being in his presence.

Because I was not allowed to hang out or have a boyfriend, I was afraid to say anything. He was also the boy that I lost my virginity to. This set the stage for my future relationships, thinking that this dysfunction was somehow normal since "everyone else was doing it."

Or, so it appeared.

This relationship resulted in my getting pregnant and having an abortion. My parents were hurt, and I am sure they felt that they had provided for me as best as they knew how. They made sure that my relationship soon ended with him.

My mom did not want me to be a young, single parent (or a single parent at all), as she knew the struggles that she had faced prior to marrying and after divorcing my stepdad. Despite their efforts, I went on to be in situation-ships and relationships with other guys, to include my son's father, during my high school career, where cheating, fighting, and promiscuity were involved.

Life was not all bad. We had fun; however, it was definitely an unstable and cracked foundation.

Over the years, I resented my mother for being overprotective. However, I understand so much more clearly now that she was a mother protecting her children, and that she was depressed since the death of her mother decades earlier. Although I did not know at the time that my mother was depressed, as we reflected on the past, we could both see the symptoms of sadness, irritability, persistent low mood, low energy, and her dislike of the holidays, especially Thanksgiving, and always being in a constant state of worry; which I would later find myself experiencing.

Depression is heavy, and I can recall feeling the thickness of dread and irritability during Thanksgiving. It was difficult for me because my birthday falls on or around that holiday. I later found out that my grandmother transitioned her life on Thanksgiving Day. I never knew why my birthday never excited me and why the holidays felt so gloomy. I now know that grief and depression were the cause.

It would come into my life later.

High school was finally over! I was so excited to begin my college career, and to be honest, get away from home; you know, the sheltered life I was living and be free, or so I thought.

I can remember the day before I left for college, I spent my last hoorah with some of my best childhood friends at a football game in September 1996, the same night that we lost the great Tupac Shakur; how can I forget.

So here I am, in my freshman year, living in an apartment because I failed to turn in my housing paperwork on time for school. My mom would always tell me, *"You going somewhere because you sho ain't staying here,"* in her beautiful Georgia accent.

What I have learned is that no matter how many places we travel, we will continue to carry around the same baggage until we become aware of the detriment and chaos it is causing in the relationships we have with ourselves, our families, careers, lovers, friends and our bodies.

"Party, party, party, let's all get wasted."

It was not long before I had met friends, gotten comfortable and was having the time of my life. Remember, I was free, but what I did not know is that I still had the baggage of not knowing how to be in a healthy relationship and not knowing my worth. In our community, some may say that this is too young to know how to be in a healthy relationship, but I disagree.

My past relationships had hard wired my mind into thinking that young men cheat and are not faithful, that having sex is just part of the relationship even if I did not really enjoy it, and that relationships consisted of drama, arguing and disappointment ultimately.

I was not sure how to handle stressful situations and often lashed out in anger—all of which was dysfunctional and wrong!

I began a situation-ship with a young man who I was head over heels for, for all of the wrong reasons. He was handsome, from the city, popular, fine as hell, an upperclassman, and had a nice car. I was fresh meat and ready!

We were having sex, and I guess getting to know each other, but not really. Although my mother warned me that sex or a baby would not keep a man and that I had failed and unhealthy relationships to prove it, I had still not connected that what I was doing was not working. It wouldn't connect until years later. Well, one day he disappeared, and the phone calls stopped. I was crushed and did not have the proper coping skills to work through the rejection.

It just felt like I could not get away from the pain of relationships, often left feeling confused.

I came across a statement in my 30's that says, "Hurt people, hurt people." It was not soon before I allowed this feeling of disappointment to translate into feelings of anger. Our egos—and the need for control that drives us—can eat away at us slowly, if not put in check. I felt abandoned and unheard.

That same week I went to visit and ended up having sex with my ex-high school sweetheart who I had not been intimate with since my situation-ship began with the upperclassmen, plus my ex-high school sweetheart had a new girlfriend. I learned later that this was dysfunctional, but remember, that is the place in which I had operated from for so many years.

I was determined not to feel vulnerable, abandoned and rejected, although that is exactly how I felt. I eventually saw my upperclassman again, and our encounters continued until summer break began.

He went home, and I went to N.C.

Over summer break, I found out that I was 19 and pregnant. Stressed and scared to tell my mom, I decided to call him and let him know. Someone else told my mom before I could. He accepted responsibility, and once fall semester kicked back, we would spend time together, and he would read to the baby in my belly. It sounds good, but by this time my self-esteem was pretty low. See, I had placed my self-esteem and happiness in my situation-ships and what I knew about them is that they didn't last; and, at some point or another, were filled with drama and disappointment.

This same year, my sophomore year, I declared Psychology as my major. I could not think of anything else I would be good at besides helping people with their problems.

Heck, I seemed to spend a lot of time dealing with my own problems and talking to my friends for hours about theirs. Choosing psychology was one of the best decisions I have made in my life. I fell in love the day I was in class, and the professor began talking about the self-fulfilling prophecy, which simply put, means that what we think becomes a reality.

I thought this was the coolest idea ever but was not sure how this thing that sounded so magical could become true, yet I wanted it. It seemed unattainable for me because I had so much trouble controlling my emotions and thoughts due to the unhealthy thinking patterns I had developed and witnessed.

It is beautiful how things come full circle, as this would later be the basis for much of the work I do with my integrative practice of counseling, spiritual coaching, yoga, and Reiki.

Being a woman who was young, pregnant and in a situationship was scary, for lack of a better word. I did know, however, that he would be there for the baby. Shortly after having my son, a paternity test showed that my high school sweetheart was my son's father. I remember that day, as I had just finished baking my upperclassman a German Chocolate cake, his favorite, and frying codfish for him.

My son was with my friend, his "Godmother" at the time.

It felt like my soul was being ripped from my body. I felt like I was in a nightmare and can remember falling to the floor screaming at the top of my lungs over and over again.

A part of me died that day—I have since then opened the door to let her (myself) live in peace—but, it was hell getting here. I remember calming down enough so that my friends would leave me be; all the while thinking about my baby, and that I had to get him and run away.

Once they were no longer hovering around me, I ran for the door, jumped in my car, and left. Upon returning home, I realize that he had gotten into my apartment and taken his things. We talked days later as he took my son and me to eat. It was also the first time I recall him telling me that he loved me and that he knew I had not done it intentionally.

I was crushed, disappointed, and rejected once again, and although the words sounded good at the moment, I was now numb and broken.

He moved away back to the city after the school year ended. I think that it devastated him as well, but he was able to go on with life, as I was the bad guy, the whore, the one that was not good enough for him; which were the things that I told myself. He never said these things.

Many may think that I did it to myself. I would have to agree wholeheartedly. I hated myself so much for this and would spend hours talking about it with my roommate. It hurt so badly, and I just wanted someone to understand how bad I hurt, how much I never meant for this to happen, and how much I loved him. My heart felt broken into tiny pieces.

I was operating on autopilot, and I know that this affected me as a mother. Guilt riddles me to this day; just not as heavy or as often, thank God. I often apologize to my son for any stress, anxiety, or sadness that my state of being brought to him, because there is no way that it could not have.

Gone untreated, it not only affects the person directly suffering but those around them as well.

I lived with this shame and self-pity throughout my stay in college and years after. My remaining college years found me in a state of embarrassment, deep sorrow, rejection, depression, anxiety, and self-medicating with *Black & Mild*s, marijuana, alcohol, cigarettes, and sex; while seeking approval from young men, who had neither true interest in me nor were emotionally available.

Although broken, I refused to fold and go home to my mother's; to the small town I had grown up in. Instead, I stayed in school, maintaining a full academic load, and being required to work or volunteer 20 hours a week to pay for childcare. This was the first time in my life that I received public assistance, food stamps, and a welfare check.

The strained relationship as a result of absence, finances, and poor communication was the theme my son's father and I had for the first 18 years of our son's life. This has improved in many ways, and little in others, over the last two years.

For the remaining years in college, I felt *less than*, overlooked, and rejected. Much of it had to do with how I felt about myself. I found out a year later that one of my best friends, who I'd known since grade school, slept with my upperclassman the night that he found out my son was not his. Here it is again, that cycle of sex, betrayal, and low self-worth.

Remember, "hurt people, hurt people" and until you uncover the root, the tree of despair, depression, low self-worth, failed relationships and anxiety will permeate like cancer in our lives.

I graduated college with a BS in Psychology and a minor in Child and Family Development and went on to teach Special Education for seven years. Then, after obtaining my Master's degree in Counseling, I worked for six years as a School Counselor. Even after college, I found myself in the cycle of turbulent, unfulfilling, emotionally and mentally draining relationships. At some point during the ride, the following feelings and themes were present: cheating, arguing, ignoring, feeling abandoned, sabotaging, and transferring what happened to me in previous relationships on to the new one, with them perhaps doing the same in return; like the self-fulfilling prophecy I mentioned earlier.

As I have done the work over the years, I realized I believe that we do the best that we can with the mental and emotional stamina we have; based on experiences we have encountered.

Although this has all been an experience and one could not have occurred without the other, I would say that my mid 30's met me in a space where I was able to begin figuring out how to love myself. This meant that I also had to get naked and see all of me; the parts that were my fault, where I hurt because of my actions and no one else's.

In turn, I have wanted to help others do the same.

It has been one hell of a journey. I am grateful that this part of my life is over, and I can now not be ashamed of those moments, but instead nurture, love, heal, and share this journey with others.

After working the obtaining my degree in counseling, I worked on my licensure to become a therapist, and then six years later became a yoga instructor. I reflect on a journal entry I wrote which reads:

"As I look back over my life, it has been good."

Our individual journeys are the vehicles that deliver us to our divine and purposed destinations. I was fortunate to hear a sermon, which included the story of John 5:5 as it speaks of a man who has been an invalid for 38 years, lying by a pool with others who were afflicted (this same year I would turn 38).

Yeshua asks the man if he wants to get well and the man gives all of the reasons why he has not been healed. Then, Yeshua loudly tells him to get up, *"Pick up your mat and walk."*

And like that, the man was healed.

This made me reflect deeper into my life. What was my mat? What does the mat signify in my life?

I believe that we often have more than one 'mat', as in therapy we know that things do not appear overnight, but have been developing for years.

In 2015, I purchased a yoga mat and began a practice I had abandoned and not cultivated years before. Not for the reason that yoga required a mat, but because I experienced the way it allowed me to come on to it feeling stressed, worried, and needing to control things, and coming off of it feeling peace, faith, and the ability to let things work out as I knew they would... and always did.

Having my son at 18-years-old take his first yoga class with me, and him coming away feeling so at ease and comfortable that he fell asleep during Shavasana, was priceless; and I am forever grateful for these experiences.

Yoga, with a combination of therapeutic approaches I have learned and practiced, as well as essential oils, scripture, acknowledging our ancestors, and other holistic and spiritual practices, has taken from being broken, wanting more in my career, spiraling out of control, anxious, depressed, over-reacting, and unable to operate in relationships, and turned me into a woman with repaired and new pieces; moving forward, accepting herself, living unapologetically, learning to give and receive love, and being open to being a student, admitting mistakes, knowing that I am still a work in progress, and that life can feel GREAT much of the time!

Through sharing my integrative counseling and yoga program, I have been able to assist individuals in their professional, romantic, and interpersonal relationships; helping my family and friends gain an understanding of themselves, to be unashamed of what they have been through, becoming better parents, lovers, friends, and bosses as they move unapologetically into their true and higher self.

There is a spring from which quietness comes. Learning to get quiet so that you can hear (divinely), I believe, is important for many in the process towards healing. Have you ever tried to solve a problem, make a decision or have an effective conversation in the midst of chaos?

If you answered *'yes,'* I would now ask, "How has that been working out for you or those involved?" For many of my friends, and the counseling and coaching clients I see, the answer is "not very well at all!" Remaining in a place of chaos makes it difficult for you to hear and truly understand your patterns of dysfunction. It is time that you heal from wounds you've been carrying around for so long.

According to the **Merriam-Webster Dictionary**, healing means: *"To make free from injury or disease; to restore."* So, getting quiet helps you to be better able to manage the chaos that could potentially spew out to others, or permeate internally through you; causing infection, which is counterproductive in the healing process. Getting quiet also provides you the opportunity to tune into yourself and to God within you to understand what direction to take, what needs healing, how to heal, how to love, how to live.

It is at the point you realize that by shifting in the opposite direction to things that feel good (instead of doing the same thing and feeling bad), that situations will begin to change for the better. Healing comes when you are able to get real, to acknowledge that you are thinking in these ways or exhibiting these behaviors.

It may mean having what feels like a difficult conversation with yourself. On this path, you learn to accept yourself for who you are, where you are and know and accept that you are a vibrational being guided by the Divine; cultivating a state of quiet, gifts you with the opportunity to hear.

Yoga helps us get quiet so that we can hear.

In earlier practices of yoga, people would sit in poses for great lengths of time, to prepare their bodies to sit in meditation.

"Prayer is talking to God.
Meditation is listening to God."
-Unknown

Yoga within the African American community is becoming more acknowledged and practiced than ever; although that number is still very small compared to our non-African American counterparts.

An estimated 2% of African American women practice yoga. The truth of this can be observed just by visiting most yoga studios and yoga teacher trainings throughout the United States.

When discussing yoga, most people of color that I converse with think yoga is only poses, or that it involves worshipping another God; which scares people.

However, yoga can be what you make it.

It can be a physical, mental, or spiritual practice. It can help lower blood pressure, help with back pain, lower stress levels, help you with feelings of anxiety and depression, improve your relationship with yourself and your loved ones, support you improving your body image, or help you open up to the infinite possibilities of the universe.

There are eight different limbs (parts) of yoga:

1. Yamas - Ethical standards and integrity
2. Niyamas - Self-discipline and spiritual observances
3. Asanas – Poses
4. Pranayama – Breathing
5. Pratyahara - Withdrawal of senses
6. Dharana – Concentration
7. Dhyana – Meditation
8. Samadhi - Connection to the Divine, bliss, or being one with the universe

You can decide which parts you would like to incorporate. Some people choose just to do the poses, and that is fine. The important thing is doing what works for you.

Practicing yoga as a student helped me realize how beneficial it would be for my clients, family, friends, and community. This was my motivation for becoming a yoga instructor; beginning as a tool to enhance the teachings and philosophies I have adopted and utilized in my life personally and as a therapist. After having the repeated feeling of peace and clarity, I knew it was something I had to share with them.

Once I became an instructor, continuing to witness the low number of African Americans taking advantage of this healing practice, the movement **Black Minds In Meditation** was birthed; the goal being to help others understand that stress, anxiety, depression, being overwhelmed, failed relationships, feeling stuck in a career, and excessive worry do not have to be their life story.

You see, the stress of life has a way of wreaking havoc on your body (physically and mentally) and your relationships (inter-personal and intrapersonal). Many of us have adopted unhealthy coping strategies in an effort to de-stress and have, unfortunately, transferred our stress and sorrow onto our families and anyone in our path.

It is my passion to help you understand how yoga and psychotherapy can help you unpack and rid yourself of the trauma that is stored in your body by embracing the mind, body, and soul connection, and as I work with individuals in the process of building better lives for themselves and their families, the one thing I have observed is the common desire to live a life of purpose and fulfillment. However, many are moving on autopilot through life... just as I was.

Many of you are experiencing blocks, either real or imagined, that are stopping the flow of infinite abundance in your lives. On the outside, you are holding things together, but on the inside, you are empty. Somewhere along the way, you have learned that this is just the way life is. Somewhere along the way, your basic needs for safety, security, survival, self-worth, or affection were altered.

Through talk therapy and specialized meditations, Reiki, breathing and sequences, you can be the facilitator of your journey as we work together to begin to unpack the parts of yourself you have been hiding, or that have been getting in your way.

If you, or someone you know, is being affected by depression, anxiety, low self-esteem, failed relationships, or any of the things I mentioned in this chapter, consider seeking the help of a professional.

You can call, or visit, the local mental health agency in your area, the behavioral health department at your local hospital, **Psychology Today** online, speak to a medical doctor for a list of providers, or look online (or in the phone book) for supportive resources.

UNFINISHED BUSINESS

By Linda Lewter, LPC

Momma said that when it was time to give birth to me, I was going *up* instead of coming down. Doctors said that she and I could have both died. Little did I know this act of retreating would be a lifelong pattern for me.

I was the sixth child born into a family of five. The oldest was a girl, four boys in between, and then me. I was called the surprise and sometimes nothing at all because no one knew that my parents had had another child. She had gone to the doctor because she thought she was having some issues with digestion and the doctor told her she was pregnant.

She would tell me the story of how excited my youngest brother and his friends were when she was coming home from the hospital with me. There had been about 15 years since a girl had been added to this family.

This would make me smile inside every time I heard it.

Then, there was the other story about how my oldest brother was upset with my mom for getting pregnant, ranting on about how they didn't need another child and how he was not going to have anything to do with me. She told me about a time she tested him one day when I was a baby by leaving me on the bed in his view, leaving the room, and secretly watching to see if he was going to let me roll off.

Luckily, he did not; instead, he watched me intensely and yelled for her when he thought I might be getting to close to the edge.

PART I

Most of my childhood memories were filled with me, mom, and church. We were either in church three to four times a week, going somewhere with the prayer band, or visiting the sick and the elderly. Momma was the first counselor (unofficially) I ever knew. She had a big personality, and it seemed someone knew her everywhere we went. She had been called to the ministry and became an Evangelist even before I was born. She was an amazing speaker.

On the one hand, momma was my role model, and on the other hand, there never seemed to be any room "for me" in the room with her because of her big overarching personality.

Dad was a quiet man of few words who I often identified with. My dad and I were close to a certain extent, more than any of my other brothers and sisters. I think this was because I was his "baby girl" as he would affectionately call me.

My mom had given birth to me during her midlife, and there was a seven-year age difference between my brother and me, next youngest siblings, and fifteen years between me and my sister, who was the oldest. I often felt like an only child, yet with the advantages of a big family all at the same time. I remember my childhood being very lonely at times, wishing I had a twin or another sibling my age to play with.

This is the time of life when people are searching for the deeper meaning of their lives. Due to my mom's involvement in the church, I often felt like an accessory that my mom had to take around with her. We spent most of the week at the church between meetings, choir rehearsals, Wednesday prayer meetings, revivals, specials services, or my mom's speaking engagements. I remember even doing my homework on the pews in the back of the church.

I felt so different as a kid because I used to watch my youngest brother do his homework in awe.

I could not wait to get homework to do, and every Sunday night, I would force my mom to read the comic strips to me. I remember her saying how she could not wait for me to be able to read the paper myself.

As a very observant child, I often absorbed everything around me like a sponge. By the time I was in elementary school, they wanted to skip me a grade ahead, but my mom refused to let them, saying she did not want them to rush me. I excelled in school and never remember my parents having to remind me to do my homework. It was my escape and way to prove my worth and make my parents proud that I had been born, even if I had been a surprise.

By the time I was an adolescent, my mom was in the benevolence phase of her life, choosing to focus on giving back to society via volunteerism, mentorship, or philanthropy.

By this time, all of my siblings were young adults and had left home, and she was always trying to help someone, even if it meant taking in a cousin to provide them something that was missing in their family of origin. Sometimes, I secretly wished I was a stranger to my mom so that she could "see me" like she was able to "see others." It seemed as if she knew exactly what to do for others, yet did not know how to help me navigate the complex insecurities she saw in me, as I sought out who I was in this family and world.

Our religion was very legalistic, prohibiting women from wearing pants or makeup or anyone to participate in "worldly activities" such as parties where there may be dancing or alcohol. Therefore, I often could not relate to my classmates in high school who I would hear talking about parties but never invited me because I was a "church girl."

I was broken hearted because my best friend told me that he had asked another girl to go to the prom because he didn't think I would go. I wanted so much to be able to go but felt that I would not know how to fit in. Not knowing what to talk about and what I would do about the dancing. It terrified me just thinking about it. I cried myself to sleep thinking about it but knew he had made the right decision. I just wasn't like the other girls. I didn't fit in.

My dad, on the other hand, seemed to be somewhere between adolescence and early adulthood for most of my life. I had always seen my dad as a hard worker and provider. However, I never knew him to ever have any strong emotions beyond joking and being playful when my mom was mad.

The differing personalities and life stages my parents were in caused many arguments, as my mom was trying to save the world, and my dad was trying to live in it. I was often caught in the middle because I only wanted both of my parents to be happy. My mom would confide and vent to me about the intimate details and frustration of her relationship with my dad, often using the relationship I had with him to manipulate him to fulfill some request that she could not seem to get through to him.

From an early age, I remember feeling helpless, listening to them argue for hours, and I thought it would be great if I could somehow get them to really hear each other and stop hurting each other emotionally.

I just wanted the arguing to stop.

I believe my mom held on to me a little tighter because I was the last one, and my mom's identity was so wrapped up in being a mother. My mom was an only child and never really got to know her dad. Her mom had died when I was five years old. Her mom had told her that she probably had a lot of kids to make up for her lack of natural siblings.

My mom would often express her frustration or disappointment that all of her children had left home.

At times, my mom and I were also in conflict due to my desires and opinions that differed from hers.

Sometimes, I wondered if she had some jealousy over the relationship between my dad and me, in the face of not having a relationship with her dad. I also knew that I needed to leave home to fully come into my own.

So, when I graduated from high school, I knew I was going away to college. Due to the sheltered life I had lived, I knew going away would be essential for my personal growth. I went to college an hour away so that I would not be too far from home. After college, I moved two hours further away to Washington DC and became a government auditor. During this tenure in my life, I was on a quest to determine who I was and to find some satisfaction in my life.

Whenever I came home to visit, I would sometimes easily be emotionally drawn back into a triangle with my parents and would quickly escape back to my life.

After moving to DC, I discovered that my oldest brother had a drug problem. He often borrowed money from me and lived with me at one point. I later learned that my helping him was only making his addiction worst. After much prayer and anguish, I had to eventually start saying no to his request for money and even picking him up from various know drug areas. One day, he called me and said that he had quit his job and needed me to pick him up.

We hung up, and he called back about twenty minutes later and asked me if I was on my way, I said, *"No, I am not."* I had decided that I could no longer support him at the risk of disappointing my family, only hoping that he would understand.

During these young adult years, I suffered some unfulfilling relationships and did a lot of soul-searching.

Through the exposure to career counseling on the job, counseling through the church and various family addiction groups that I attended to support my brother, I learned that the very thing that I had run away from continued to be present with me because an external resolution could not fix the problem.

Internal reprogramming was necessary.

I started to have an unchaining pull to return home to my parents that I wrestled with for years. I often sympathized with my mom not having any siblings, even though she had cousins that had been raised like her sisters. I would test the waters by visiting for a week or more, but the timing never felt quite right.

However, when I returned home to DC, I would still feel the pull because my mom had started showing signs of dementia and complications managing her diabetes.

I decided to sell my house and move into an apartment so that I would not have any ties keeping me when the timing was right. Something was telling me that I needed to go back in order to move forward.

Shortly after the 9/11 tragedy in New York, I took a leave of absence under the Family and Medical Leave Act of 1993 due to one of my niece's diagnosis of Lymphoma. She had been sick for about a year and had lost a baby girl in the midst of many transfers from hospital to hospital and now had found herself in a home in Northern Virginia that took patients with a breathing tube. My niece had just turned 30 but was in a comatose state, and it was unknown to us whether she even knew it.

We would continue to talk to her, and I would read her poetry during my visits with her. Within two weeks of her relocation, she passed away. After seeing how this had weighed on my sister and considering the aging of my parents and my mom's illness, the timing felt right, and I made a move back home to Virginia.

I remember talking to the Assistant Inspector General at the Department of Education where I was employed as a GS 13 at that time, and she told me to take the leave, go home, and I could return to my good government job.

With the weight of both the 9/11 event and watching my niece come to the close of her life, I decided that I did not want to live a "what if" life. It was all or nothing for me, and I wrote a letter of resignation and started my journey home.

PART II

So here it was, the summer of 2002, when I found myself back, not only in Virginia but in my parent's house. Even though I had processed in my head all the reasons why I needed to do this, I felt as if I was in the birthing process again; *going the wrong way.*

Seeds of doubt and self-consciousness began to be planted whenever I played the mental tapes of what I thought others would say and how I would be judged about leaving my job and returning home. Again, it felt like I was going the wrong way, now my days were filled with watching *Little House on the Prairie* and Westerns while making sure I was in the house by the time the street lights came on.

I was back in the 12th grade.

I often reminded myself of all the confirmations I had received through career counseling, individual counseling and support groups that had helped me to see glimpses of who I could be. I was 38 and figured I was young enough to start over, thinking that I could return to D.C. financial status in just five years. My mom was 78 and dad 77, and my mom was facing issues with diabetes, high blood pressure, heart issues, cholesterol, glaucoma, cataracts, and now showing signs of dementia. My dad had high blood pressure, yet was still pretty fit, still riding his bike occasionally.

He was now retired, but working a small part-time job to have something to do and stay out of my mom's way.

My first task, or so I thought, was to whip my parent's diet into shape by getting rid of all the fried foods and overcooked greens to assist my mom in managing her diabetes. I volunteered to cook dinner one night and broke out my healthy recipe of baked fish and vegetables seasoned with Mrs. Dash, and a sugar-free cake.

I had fixed my parents' plates with a proud glimmer in my eye, anticipating that they were going to be so delighted to have a health-conscious, but tasty meal.

I couldn't wait for the reviews.

Mom ate some of her fish but picked at the vegetables. Dad managed to eat most of his. I asked my mom "How was it?" She stated, "I like my fish fried and the vegetables needed to be cooked a little more." She went on to explain that food was one of the pleasures that, in the midst of the many changes in her life, she was going to hold on to and eat whatever she wanted to. She wanted food that was reminiscent of the days of old.

Over time, I made a few other unsuccessful attempts, but I started to resent this attitude, saying to myself, "Look at all I have sacrificed to come down here to help them, and it's not even appreciated." I took a step back and said to myself "I guess she is right, who am I to enter their space and change everything?"

I felt defeated and must have subconsciously thought *if you can't beat them, join them*, so I gave in to the fried chicken, fish, grease, gravy, and pork-seasoned vegetables with a scoop of ice cream and assorted cakes nightly. Yes, I had officially accepted my invitation to the pity party.

With my new curfew of O'dark:30, my social life took a hit. It was a Friday night, and I was sitting at home watching **TV land** with my parents. I thought to myself, *I know I came home to help, but I can't go out like this.*

My M.O., when moving to a new area, was always to establish myself with a good church first. Well, I was still a member of the church I had mostly grown up in and would take my mother there regularly when she felt up to it. However, I had gotten a taste of the big city and the "mega-church" life where something was going on for all age groups. I had been a part of young missionary groups, single ministries, small groups, choirs, and missionary trips at various churches in DC and missed all the activities.

I loved my home church because it is where I got my foundation and found true salvation, but I felt everything was the same as when I had left in 1983, and now it was 2003.

Don't get me wrong; sameness can be good because the word of God does not change. Yet, I was longing for more, so I started exploring churches in the area that possessed more progressive ministry options. It also got me out the house after dark because my mom didn't mind you being out at night if it was church related.

My sister had been the only one still in our hometown with my parents. After seeing her go through a devastating year with my niece, "Somebody is going to have to come back to help with mama and daddy at some point" kept ringing in my ear. My sister, the oldest and fifteen years my senior, was only one of six who had never left our hometown.

I was five years old and a flower girl in my sister's wedding, having grown up more with her daughters than her.

One of her daughters described us as being total opposites. She became a registered nurse; I became an accountant. She got a car and learned to drive while in college, I was driving from the age of 13 and drove every chance my dad would let me, getting my learner's permit just shy of my 16th birthday, and a car in the 11th grade.

While she went to a local college and never left the area, I went to a school an hour away, got a job two more hours away, and after that I stayed away for 15 years. She got married right out of college and started a family, I never got married and traveled across the US extensively with some international travel mixed in. She was very passive with my parents and in her relationships. I was very vocal with both my parents and the most aggressive out of all the children.

Needless to say, we saw things differently when it came to the care of my parents and their aging issues, and even had a different relationship with them. I was very avoidant at times because I didn't want to ruin the potential of a relationship with her that I always longed for but never had.

On the social front, most of my friends who had stayed local after high school had settled into the local culture of getting a "good job," which meant it was military or government related and offered long haul retirement for the kids, the picket fence, and all that comes with that. I did have one friend, Pamela Jones, who must have sensed what I was going through because she, even though we had gone away to college together, had moved back home to live the dream, she always would reach out and pull me into her family activities. She is a lifer and will never know how her kindness affected me during that time of transition.

Because I was the youngest (never the baby) of six, I always was in the pursuit of proving my worth and measuring up to them.

This created a sense of independence in me where I felt that I always had to carry my weight.

Due to the over-nurturing environment at my parent's house, along with mine and their regressions back to days of old, I knew I needed to get my own space. I tried on some quick jobs just to continue to bring in some income to cover my expenses and not have to be dependent on my parents.

After a short stint with retail, substitute teaching, and selling Cutco knives, like the children of Israel, I came to my senses and said, "I better go back into accounting. At least with that, I am out of these labor-intensive fields."

After discovering that the local paper, *The Virginian Pilot*, was hiring, I applied. I was successful at securing an accountant position, leaving my parent's house, and moving into an apartment across the street from my job so I could walk to work. Here I was, doing what was comfortable again. I feared I would only end up right back at this point feeling empty, hopeless without passion for a job to which I felt enslaved. I decided to explore my passion for counseling and enrolled full time in the graduate program at Regent University.

The only thing I knew is that I was now following a calling and that where God gives vision, he also provides provision.

The next two years were filled with wonder for me.

We had to form cohorts, which is essentially a group of students designated to help you practice your counseling techniques. Daniall Foskey and Janice Johnson were included in my cohort. I figured this would be fun, but little did I know the surgery that was about to begin, with me being the patient.

After leaving home and moving to D.C., I was well aware that I was in search of something. This had led me to individual counseling, support groups, career counseling, and mentorship, where I was mentored by the inspector general of one of my government positions.

I thought I had a pretty good understanding of what my issues were both professionally and personally. The one thing I remembered one of my instructors saying is that it was crucial to do the work on yourself during this period so that you do not show up in the room with your client, and that if you do show up, you can quickly identify it and address the situation. I made the decision to let it all hang out.

This went against the grain of everything I had been taught from the African American perspective, whether consciously or subconsciously of *"what happens in this house, stays in this house."* Also, I was aware of the cultural history of African Americans not being able to trust the system because of the inability of those outside our culture to identify with our perspective because of the two faces that the African American often has to portray for mere survival.

Also, there is a fear in our community of showing any signs of weakness for fear it will be held against you by those in authority or you will be stereotyped and categorized when you are so desperately trying to stand out and prove your worth. We all took an oath of confidentiality, which is the same confidentiality that all counselors take when working with clients. This process allowed me to, once again, go back and process things from the womb for a rebirthing that I never imagined.

I noticed a release in me of expectations, hurts, and longings that I was still holding on to, which resulted in me being able to begin to show up toward my family with more patience, long-suffering, gentleness, and not seeking the fulfillment of my own needs. I had come back home to make some changes, but the changes were now happening in me.

I was just getting into the groove of things with my classwork, practicum, and a mindless job I had taken at the school library, to keep some gas in my car, when we got a call that my oldest brother was sick. We had come to find out that he was in the last stages of colon cancer. He had taken sick and had to have emergency surgery.

After getting through the surgery and stabilized, he decided that he did not want any further surgeries, stating that God would heal him if it was meant to be and asked my parents if he could come home. I had to explain to my mom, who was now showing more signs of dementia, the gravity of what he was asking. Whether she understood it or not she said, as she had always told any of us, "You can come home if you can't go anywhere else."

I think this situation allowed my sister and me to bond like we never had before. With the health of my mom declining, my parents would not be able to care for him, and that responsibility fell on the two of us. I became his champion in all things natural, exploring each natural remedy we learned about, and even finding a health resort that treated a number of illnesses through diet changes. Without being able to live at the resort, and have space, there was a daunting task to maintain the rigorous diet. It was simply too little, too late.

It was on a Tuesday, November 15, 2005, when he departed. But, the day before, I spent the day with him at the hospital.

We were visited that day by family and friends.

One of my cousins, who was a minister, came by at my brother's request and had communion with him, and we sang old familiar hymns. I sat in awe thinking how proud and at peace I was, being able to see this process of my brother making peace within himself spiritually. My mind went back to when my brother had come home from his service as a Marine in the 70's and how he had closed himself off from his childhood beliefs and held a lot of anger regarding the injustices that he saw in society. I was afraid of him because of the coldness he displayed toward me. I was the little sister that he never wanted and never got to know.

Now here we were. I was given the honor to be a part of his last days and have an opportunity to serve him in this crucial stage in his life. As the sun went down and all of the guests left, he asked me if I would stay the night with him because he was scared. My heart dropped within me. I felt closer to him at this very moment than I ever had in my entire life.

The child in me wanted to drop everything and stay at his side, but I was in the midst of finals, with an exam and paper due the next day. I had to make a choice. I assured him of the support from the nurses that were only a buzzer away, of the host of angels, and of God himself, all of whom were there with him.

The next day when I called him, my brother answered the phone, yet seemed a little disoriented. He seemed to be talking to someone and said to me, *"They're here."*

I said, "*Oh, the nurses are in the room?*" and proceeded to tell him where they could find his items for his morning care routine and breakfast. He then said, "*The nurse is not here yet.*"

I figured he must have still been tired or dreaming and told him to go ahead and get some rest and I loved him and would check on him later.

It was later that evening when I called to check on my mom that she said she didn't know what was going on but my sister and a cousin who was helping to take care of my brother had been called to the hospital. I immediately got off the phone with her and called my sister. My sister confirmed that the doctors had called and said my brother was passing.

I was frantic, wondering why my sister had not called me.

Of all the nights I could have loaned my car to a classmate to go to the library, I chose that one. I called her, and when she returned, I drove to the hospital, which was twenty minutes away. When I arrived, the bed was empty. My sister said he had just died and they had taken him to the morgue. I asked her for the details: Was he in pain? Did he say anything? She stated that after he passed there was a peaceful look about him.

I took solace in that.

When I later spoke with some of my fellow counselors, they helped me process the irony of me and my brother's relationship and the incredible gift that I had been given. And, I completed coursework for my Master's in Counseling/Psychology in the month following his passing.

The loss of my brother hit my mother hard. She could not talk about him without breaking down. I began to see her health steadily decline. Initially, I became angry with her at times and lectured her on things she should and should not do and eat to help with some of the challenges that diabetes and a sedentary life-style was causing. I did not like the thoughts and feelings that I was having, and sometimes I resented my siblings for not being more involved in the care of my mom. I was forced to start educating myself on the issues of dementia and Alzheimer's. I later came to realize that I was going through the stages of grief as I was losing pieces of my mom right before my very eyes.

In the midst of this process, pivotal advice came from Janice, from my cohort. She said to me in so many words that I needed to give the care of my mom over to someone else so that she can maintain her dignity and so I can start enjoying my visits with her instead of resenting them.

This was a turning point for me. Although this process was not without challenges, it was by far the best advice I could have gotten. The last years with my mom became a journey of helping her to look back over her life to reminisce about her greatest accomplishments. I compiled a DVD that included her life as a young adult, mother and husband, and minister. This sparked a lot of fond memories for her, especially since the long-term memory is more intact in a person suffering from dementia or Alzheimer's.

Sometimes we had to be careful when showing her that DVD because she would stay in that period, since her short-term memory was spotty, and would get in a frantic state saying that she had to go somewhere and preach. It would take a while to settle her down to the here and now.

For my mom's birthday September 25, 2012, I decided to send out invitations to family and friends of my mom's asking them to send me a card or letter stating the impact she had on their life with a picture.

You see, it was getting hard for my mom to recognize voices on the phone. We were flooded with cards and letters that culminated in a book I presented to her on her birthday and reviewed every letter and picture with her over the next months. I remember her saying after one of our review sessions, "I guess I have done some good in the world."

To which I replied, *"Yes, Ma. You have indeed."*

Sometime after that, during a doctor's visit where I was accompanying her, I remember her sharing a story with me that I had never heard. She said to me, "Did I ever tell you how you got here?" I had heard her tell of how I was a surprise many times but figured I would play along. I said, "no, how?"

She then told this story:

> "Well, it had been some years since I had a baby, and your brother was getting bigger and starting school when I said to myself, *I need another baby and preferably a little girl.* So, I prayed and asked God to let me have one more child... and then we had you."

That day was a rebirthing for me of sorts. I felt something stand up inside of me; like, I don't have to apologize for my existence anymore. I belong here.

The days that followed became more challenging due to complications from diabetes. We had to have one of her toes amputated and was now looking at a second toe or perhaps foot, and I remember driving from my parents' house back to my condo and crying out to God that she did not deserve this after how she had tried to live her life for Him.

Around the beginning of March 2013, my mom fell and sprained her ankle. A week later, the doctor pulled me aside and said she was at the end of life. On Friday, March 8, 2013, my mom took her final breath in a room full of family and friends, with my dad holding her left hand and me holding her right. The last thing I whispered to her was, "Ma, we are all going to be alright. We are all grown now, and you have taught us how to live successful lives. Take your rest."

The years that followed my graduation, I continued to grow professionally and personally as I continued to stay in counseling in one form or another, be it self-help books, support groups, individual counseling, grief counseling, mentoring, personal development programs, or coaching.

At some point, I finally began to see and understand that counseling is not a one-time occurrence, but a lifelong process of being able to step outside of yourself and gain the perspective of an objective party into the true progressions of your life. It allows you to go from living life in black and white to living in color by adding all the details and nuances that the color palette brings.

This happens through the use of getting in touch with the subconscious, labeling, connecting, and processing the events of our lives from a 3D perspective in a safe and therapeutic setting, which allows you to go back to some of the most painful and vulnerable times in your life only to be propelled forward to unlimited distances.

This has been the trajectory of my life from my very birthing process to this present moment, and I am sure, of moments to come.

"Where no counsel is, the people fall:
but in the multitude of counselors there is safety."
-Proverbs 11:14

IF YOU COULD READ MY MIND

By Reginald V. Cunningham, Sr., EdD

"If you could read my mind, you'd be in tears.
If you could feel what I feel, you'd be in pain.
If you could see what I see, you'd want to be blind.
If you had a heart just like mine, you'd wish forever and a day
that you would never have been born into this world of grey."
-Unknown

Finding yourself lost in a world you thought you knew can be a desolate place, leaving you hopelessly in search of just one more—yea, just one more—to rescue you, while simultaneously planning on how and where to get the next.

It lurks on you ever so slowly, cunningly wrapping its full armor so tightly around you that you find it hard to take your next breath. It's grip altering your being into something you can no longer recognize. Whispering at first, but then crescendoing so loudly that all you want to do is run and hide. Losing the respect of family and loved ones causes you to shrink shamefully into a black hole of utter despair; a ceaseless cycle towards the pit of a catastrophic hell.

And, even then, the thought to just end it all is not foreign.

Now, alone and isolated from everyone and everything that you've learned is right in the world, you ask the question, *"Lord, why me?"*

The answer? *"Why NOT me?"*

My name is Reggie, and I'm an addict!

The "come up" for me was easy. My brother, my only sibling, and I were born and brought up in an environment that afforded us pretty much the best of everything—two hard-working parents who gave us everything we needed, and most of all, everything we wanted.

I remember Sunday dinners, where the four of us sat around the table eating together after church. I remember being dressed in some of the finest clothes. I remember going skating and to the movies regularly with my neighborhood friends. I remember my dad sitting in the bleachers watching me at baseball games, saying, *"Hit that ball boy!"*

I remember talks with my mother about the importance of school and making excellent grades, which I did throughout my parochial years. Actually, that wasn't a choice; getting straight A's was the cardinal rule in my house, or else...

I also remember road trips to the South to visit my extended family. And, I remember Christmas. We had great Christmases. The living room would be engulfed with all that we had asked for and more. When I take an inventory of my life, I had it so much easier than those around me. However, all of this 'life goodness' came with certain expectations: like love and respect for my parents and other adults, stellar educational accomplishments, and a thorough understanding of right and wrong. Yet, with all the advantages of a privileged upbringing, I fell.

The "come down" for me was a slow, but devastating ride. I didn't even see it coming. I think it was around the time I was in the eighth or ninth grade. Having become this nerd of a person, I found myself in the shadows of those I longed to emulate. I had always been this chubby kid, often full of shame and angry at my size and appearance.

Although I always wore nice clothes, I didn't look like other "brothers," such as Willie, Phil, and of course, *Pretty Tony*.

Yes, I began measuring my appearance to that of males I thought looked better than me, always dressed to the "9's". I started hanging with what we called back in the day, "the *IN* crowd" — those who smoked Kool cigarettes, drank beer, and soon, those who smoked weed. I wanted to feel like I belonged... you know, normal. I'll have to say that I did pretty good, being able to mix with a certain group that gave me that feeling of belonging.

At least I thought I did.

By the time I was in high school, especially after my parents had given me my first car, I was *IN*. Friday night dances at Mizpah and Bradfield Community Centers were nights I lived for. My friends and I would always be able to get beer and wine before going out, and at least one of us always had some of that good shit to smoke.

We'd walk in, and everybody could tell we were high. Most times you could smell the weed on us because we had just finished smoking. Drinking and getting high on weed soon became the norm. At least it's what I thought everyone did and was expected to do. This journey of my "come down" slowly, but steadily, progressed and I found myself advancing my high to snorting cocaine almost daily, eventually finding myself with a pipe in my mouth.

My whole world literally started to go up in smoke.

Then, I was well into adulthood, a college graduate, a military veteran, and divorced. I was now living in D.C., employed, but working and living a lie and a life in the grips of active addiction. I had become a "crack-head"—a title I refused to claim in the beginning. See, I believed that I was different from the stereotypical addict: jobless, living on the street or from house to house, dirty and smelly, basically, the scum of the earth. I remember sitting in the crack house with other crackheads, bragging about the fact that I had graduated from college.

Nevertheless, after finding myself on paydays anxiously waiting for the clock to strike 4:30 so that I could cash my check and head to the hood to begin my cycle of destruction, what else could I call myself?

Especially after finding myself in a hospital room after a weekend drug run which resulted in contracting such a bad case of pneumonia that the doctors informed me that I could be dead within six months.

Yeah, these pains were at the time unbearable.

Following were the wasted years of getting high, which stifled my academic and professional success. In time, I didn't have a place to call my own. No job and no means of income; depending on close friends to come to my rescue. And that one day, while walking up to a curb of a very busy intersection, I seriously contemplated walking right out into the moving traffic. I had become something that never in my wildest dreams could I have imagined… totally lost.

I can admit it now. I had become one of them. A person whose life had completely changed from that which I had once known, finding it comfortable to be in this strange new environment, sitting around a table in roach-infested public housing. Hell, I looked forward to it. And, the people there looked forward to me coming around because I was the type of addict that when I get high, I go all the way. Buying and sharing with everyone so that I could feel a sense of belonging and to feel big and important.

That monkey was riding my back fiercely. So much so, that everything dear to me went in the pipe. I had begun to live to get high and had become so naive I didn't understand the manipulation of the drug, and the manipulation of the people with which I surrounded myself.

Once, when I was forced to return to Ohio because I had nowhere else to go, I moved back to my family home. My dad had moved on and was living in a nearby city, but came to check on the house from time to time. One time, I remember him stopping at the door as he began to leave, looking back at me with total disgust, saying, *"I hate I let you bogart your way back into this house."*

I could feel the anger, but most importantly, the hurt that exuded from him. His son, his prodigal son, the one he had so many high hopes for, had fallen to this.

Active addiction is a dangerous life, and there are only three outcomes for a person in its grip: jails, institutions, and death. I barely escaped the confines of jail. I did, however, find myself in various institutions, which marked only failed attempts at rehab. But, I experienced a spiritual death so severe that it almost killed me. Soon, my bottom became apparent when I found myself jobless, homeless, and hopeless.

Let me emphasize no one has in his or her mind the dream of growing up and becoming an addict. Drinking alcohol and smoking weed was fun in the beginning; it was how we socialized, how we had fun, how we felt a sense of "belonging." As time passed, it became dishearteningly apparent that my drug use had advanced to the point of using just to feel normal, and more importantly, to escape the feelings I had buried inside me... feelings of inadequacy, low self-esteem, anger, sadness, regret, and a host of others.

No one could have told me that one day I would resort to a substance to take away pain I had not even begun to acknowledge. Such as, the pain of cancer robbing me of a longer life with my mother, my rock, when I was only 22 years old and a junior at Tennessee State University.

Right before the Thanksgiving Holiday, I had just pledged my fraternity, Kappa Alpha Psi, and was preparing to go home. I didn't know that she was in the hospital. She had never complained of anything more than a cold, so when I visited her, I didn't take it that seriously. This was *MOM*, and I told myself that she would be alright. And when I returned home for the Christmas break, she was back to herself. Or, at least I thought she was, not recognizing there was a monster eating at her insides.

By mid-January of the next year, I received a call from my brother telling me that she was back in the hospital and very sick. I knew it must be serious because her two brothers were already on their way from Alabama to pick me up and bring me home. We arrived in the wee hours of the morning, and I asked to be taken directly to the hospital.

As I approached her room, it was like something from a TV show or movie. The lights were on dim, and all I could see were machines with flashing lights and beeping sounds.

If you could have read my mind at that moment, you would understand I felt like a little boy—scared to death. Even more devastating was the belief she didn't know who I was. But, I realize it must have been because of medications they were pumping into her still body. My cousin told me that she had a form of liver cancer that had progressed rapidly. She told me that Mom was not going to live, but that she would get well enough to go home.

'Til this day, I don't know where my mind went. All I remember was my body sliding down the side of the wall, trying to embrace a pain I had never experienced.

Mom did begin to show signs of improvement, enough to be taken out of ICU and into a private room. It's funny now, but while still on pain medication, she was able to utter to me, *"You better take your ass back to school!"*

Two days later, that's exactly what I did. Those were the last words I heard my mother say. A few weeks after, my dad called and told me I needed to go straight to the airport, *"Your ticket is already paid for. Come home now."*

Upon getting there, she had sunk into a coma. I could tell by her breathing that she must have been in unbearable pain. She never recovered, and of course never came home, at least not to her earthly one.

Following her death, if you could have read my mind, you would have known that I struggled internally. I wrestled with the idea that because while growing up, I had entertained thoughts of what it would be like without my mom, I believed her death was somehow my fault. Never in my wildest imagination did I ever think that she would leave me so soon.

Then, there was also the pain of growing up with a father who, although providing every necessity and want, never uttered the words *I love you* or showed any of the bonding emotions I had witnessed between my peers and their fathers.

My dad was a very hard-working man—that I can never take from him. But, my dad was also someone who had suffered his own pain and disappointments from his dad and his upbringing. Learning just how poor he and his siblings grew up, I knew he wanted the best for me, and the only way he knew how to demonstrate that desire was to raise me with an iron fist. I don't believe he was always that way with me, at least from birth until around my third year in school.

Those years are now quite vague though.

After moving into a new neighborhood, one that was probably at the time dominated by non-black families, I remember being friends with a white boy down the street from us, and I still remember his name: Mark Smith. I visited him almost daily. It was there that I discovered a different family dynamic; one where the father played an active role in the family function.

You know... the kind you see on TV.

In my time, that kind of family was called "Leave It to Beaver" types of families. Yes, I'm a witness, they did actually exist. So, as I got older, the memory of Mark's family remained etched in my brain, and I soon began to question my mom, *"Why doesn't Dad love me?"* While she tried to convince me that he did love me, her words just fell on deaf ears because his actions didn't demonstrate 'love.'

Those talks would often leave me in tears. His voice, when telling me to do something, or even asking a question, was always with extreme aggression and anger. It both saddened and angered me, as he was rarely that aggressive with my brother who is six years younger than me. At that time, he appeared to favor my brother over me, which, in my mind, confirmed my thinking.

Was it because I was never interested in the normal activities that most boys engage in? Although I was one helluva baseball player, I didn't play sports like football or basketball, and these were the only times I felt his interest in what I was doing.

Yet, I was extremely musically skilled, singing in choirs and playing instruments. I was an awesome artist, being able to draw almost anything.

When I look back on it now, I was being a spoiled brat. I was sixteen and had gotten my driver's license. All of my friends were getting mini bikes, which was the thing to have at the time. I wanted one so bad... but he refused to get me one. However, he bought one for my brother. I couldn't for the life of me understand why. To me, the fact that he had given me a car wasn't reason enough to purchase my brother one and not me.

Okay, I admit it, I was spoiled. Materialistically that is, and felt I deserved one just the same. Again, somewhere in the crevices of my mind, I knew my dad loved me, but it was times like this that I questioned it.

As I prepared for my freshmen year at Tennessee State University, I could tell he was excited. I remember hearing him telling my mom to make sure I had everything I needed. But, his attitude toward me never changed.

I happened to be home from school when my grades for the semester arrived. I was enrolled in 21 credits hours, and of course, that was an extreme load. I also had a work-study job but was able to earn all A's and one B, making the Dean's list.

Man, was I proud of myself.

As I stood behind my dad at the kitchen table while he looked at my grades, he didn't blink. He just handed me my grades over his shoulder and said, *"You can do better."* I was crushed, once again. Yes, the fact of the matter is I could have made straight A's, but damn. Although he continued to pay for my college education, I grew emotionally distant from him, and it would take years for me to finally be able to shake the resentful feelings I developed toward him.

I am happy to report today that we have an awesome relationship. He witnessed my downfall firsthand, and I realize it hurt him terribly. I hear from family how proud he is of me, my being a doctor and all. I laugh to myself sometimes because if I don't call my dad at least every other week, I get a call from him saying in that voice of aggression that I remember so well, *"What you doin? You ain't called!"*

The difference today is *I KNOW* it's nothing but love.

If you could read my mind, you'd grasp how extremely difficult it was for me to begin to understand how my addiction was my way of coping with the ghosts I kept hidden. Oh, the many masks we take on to shield our truths from the world around us. The masks that hide insecurity, low self-esteem, diminished worth, hating the body you're born in, anger, and resentment.

These, and many more, are the feelings and emotions I would not dare reveal. And I can't ignore the regret I developed. Regret that the one person who now means the world to me, the one I'd give my life for, I had neglected.

That was my son! He was only three at the time. After his mom and I separated and eventually divorced, the devastation my departure had on him was enormous and worsened in the years to come.

The ghosts and demons in my mind grew, and as they did, so did my drug and alcohol use. For approximately 15 years of his life, I was what every man does not like to be called... "a deadbeat dad!" Yeah, I loved him to the moon and back, but I was nowhere in the picture; at least, not his. In those 15 years, I was absent and provided no monetary support to his mother for his welfare, nor to her for that matter. I think I may have seen him all of five or six times during those years.

As he got older, he eventually came to harbor extreme anger and resentment towards me for the hardship I placed on him and his mother.

At the same time, I tried to come back into his life, playing the role of his father. He had already graduated high school and completed a year at Howard University when he came to live with me. He gave me a letter he had written which emphasized his feelings about me. Even though I was clean and sober when discovering this, if you could read my mind, you'd know this almost killed me.

The feelings he described were so clear and true that it pierced my soul deeply. He told me in the letter that due to my absence, he was often asked about his father. He would make up the story that I was working in some top-secret government job and had to be away. He told me how he hated his name, being named after me because it was a reminder of my absence. He told me that due to my void, it was difficult for him to form healthy relationships with men.

There is no doubt that if you could have watched me as I read the words on that paper, even as dark as I am, you would have seen the blood flush through my body. I am just so thankful that by that time I had a solid foundation, through therapy and drug rehab, I had developed effective coping strategies to see me through this.

Reconciling my relationship with my son was not easy. I know he has forgiven me, but I'll have to admit I am often haunted by that fact that because of my absence we never had the opportunity to develop that father/son bond that I wish for today. Even now, there are times when I am jealous of the relationship he has with his mom and how he celebrates her, particularly on social media.

If you could read my mind, you'd see how depressed I can sometimes get, just wanting my son to come to me and say, "Dad I need to talk to you about this or that" or "I need your advice on whatever, etc." There are times when I think that because of my absence and the years I drowned myself in drugs, that he doesn't value my views on life.

Even more disheartening, I don't have a right to even offer advice or teach him anything. Who do I have to blame but myself? I do have the hope that he sees the changes I've made in my life and possibly looks up to me in some form of fatherly way. I am, however, grateful for the relationship we have built over recent years and I believe it grows stronger every day.

One would think that once a person has been able to conquer years of addictive behaviors, that life would magically become wonderful. Nevertheless, *if you could read my mind*, you'd see that the committee in my mind just would not adjourn. I still had to contend with the memories that mean something and the ones that don't, leaving me like a box full of darkness yet still having to deal with the root of my pain. My addiction alone was just a symptom of a larger picture that covered the canvas of my life.

Kid Cudi said it best in his chilling words on social media before checking himself into rehab:

> *"If I didn't come here, I would have done something to myself. I simply am a damaged human swimming in a pool of emotions every day of my life. There's a raging violent storm inside of my heart at all times."*

When I did a thorough self-inventory of every aspect of my life, it revealed the multiple layers of emotions with which I had not learned to cope. When you've developed the courage to search within, taking that next step of seeking professional help continues to be a difficult and scary path to take. You might ask the question, *"What was going to therapy like for you?"* The only answer I can offer is this: "it was like throwing up my insides!" And, as I began the process of finding and redefining myself, I began to understand just how much pain and turmoil I had locked up inside me.

Historically, as black men, we are taught that it's weak to be emotional or talk about our feelings. And you cannot ignore the proverbial, "Boys don't cry!" We've heard this our entire lives from the media, peers, and even family members. What's sad is that these sentiments continue to reverberate loudly to this day. Growing up as a child, I never witnessed the spectrum of varying emotions from my father or from any male figure for that matter.

What I did hear is this: "Only sissies cry."

The ideas which support this type of hyper-masculine expectations are what many of our young boys are forced to adopt, which is supposed to translate into them demonstrating strength and so-called *manliness*.

Denzel Washington's Oscar-winning drama, *"Fences,"* based on the Tony Award and Pulitzer Price-winning 1987 play by August Wilson, strongly depicts hyper-masculine behavior, which poignantly portrays how Black men have come up through the ranks of masculinity, mortality, dreams, hopes, plans, mothers, family, commitment, betrayal, duty, dissatisfaction, and life itself—in fact, even more so the meaning of life itself.

When "life," as you would have it, turns its back on us, for whatever reason, seemingly robbing us of our aspirations, hopes, and dreams, more times than not we lock up those feelings and emotions inside us and throw away the key, leaving us ignorant and incapable of how to cope with life.

How does one sum up the meaning behind the experiences and add definition to their reality? It is this undercurrent depression that finds itself rooted in the economic schema that many black men battle. We hide this secret underneath an assortment of layers, including an exaggerated bravado, drug and alcohol abuse, misdirected anger, and other forms of destructive behaviors.

Fantastical illusions are also a tool that is deployed to cope with the humbling realities of an often-marginalized existence. We also hide this secret, particularly as a "baby-boomer," because these types of crises were not acknowledged during our upbringing. Breaking the taboo of depression in black men is, and has been, at the forefront of generational struggles for decades.

I had no idea of it then, but depression had been a constant demon for the better part of my life as I am sure that young readers of my words will be particularly surprised to hear. However, like most black men, it's something we just do not talk about. Besides, why increase identity stigmatization? Why give society another reason to question our ability? Why in the world would I be this vulnerable? I'll suffer over here in silence and keep my mental illness between me and God.

But, if we don't take action and take action now, as black men, we perpetuate the ongoing negative stigmas society has already attached to us.

Our silence is killing us.

Being black today, as well as historically, is linked to various stereotypes and incorrect narratives. The stereotypes that we are strong and fast are ones we can mostly identify with. However, the problem exists in the fear that comes with being black—those subtle, and sometimes overt forms of microaggressions when a white person may cross the street and sometimes single out a black boy or man within a group. I have personally witnessed white people obviously feeling uneasy when standing next to them on the subway. In these situations, white America continues to remind us that we are *less than*.

The onslaught of police killings due to the rash profiling of black men like Michael Brown, Trayvon Martin, and a host of others—who were assumed to be dangerous and the source of conflict has played a major role in black people's vulnerability to mental health stress, and more importantly, in their refusal to seek treatment.

Even after the many protests around the country following the senseless killing of African Americans, and after the acquittal of the men in blue, we as black Americans are left reeling with emotions. Whether personally witnessing these events, or by witnessing them through social media and the news, these events are traumatizing.

All across the country, where these killings take place, Black America experienced the psychological toll it places on the community. This "race-based" trauma black people often face, results in them being increasingly susceptible to mental health conditions that need attention. There is clear, empirical research that demonstrates how racism can adversely affect mental health in both direct and indirect ways. It can inflict psychological trauma, create unfavorable socioeconomic conditions which increase the risk of psychiatric disorders, and lead to negative feelings of self-worth and overall well-being.

The problem is this: most African Americans, particularly black men, either are unable to identify the correlation between racism and mental illness or in most cases, deny their true emotions for fear of being considered to have a mental illness.

Today, we struggle against this known traumatic event called racism because it seems no matter which way we turn we are reminded of our second-class citizenship, which is ultimately damaging to the psyche.

Because of this, we as black men are left to figure it out. We don't have time to be sad or depressed because we have too many things we have to deal with right now. We have consistently tended to stuff things down, hold it in, and keep moving forward until something creates an acute crisis in the individual, and they're forced to have an intervention of some sort with an institution because of a type of psychotic break.

We don't have time to go to therapy—something we have considered a "white thing." White people can afford to be human, be vulnerable, and seek mental health care.

Black people can't.

Furthermore, the mental health field has been and still is today dominated by white mental health providers with minimal to no knowledge of the Black experience in America.

While working on my master's degree, I asked a professor, who is black, "Should blacks only seek services from black clinicians?" She responded by saying that neither race nor gender should be a factor for anyone seeking mental health services. I believed that for a long time.

I have, after years in the field, come to believe that is not necessarily true. The fact is that most, if not all, educational curriculum neglects to discuss the African American experience. Yes, there is "a" course in Multicultural Counseling, but how does one learn of the Black experience through one course, from a text-book that is limited to one chapter on the African American population?

To that end, our profession is grounded in theory—a theory that was rooted primarily in white America. Although these various theories and therapeutic modalities have relevance today, a clinician cannot have a solid sense of the Black experience through education alone. Also, they must seek ongoing individual work. To void themselves of their own biases, blacks seeking therapy and counseling services stand the chance of not receiving quality services and the possibility of further trauma.

As the paradigm of people of color taking the risk of seeking professional help for the ills we suffer increases, so does the demand for qualified professionals.

Therefore, it is critical that both black and white students in the counseling field obtain training to address the dynamics of racism, historical baggage, and the experiences of black people. For far too long, black men have suffered in silence, not even aware of the symptomatology of mental illness, and its relation to substance abuse, domestic violence, anger issues, abandonment, etc.

We are undoubtedly in need of effective ways of ridding ourselves of the emotional baggage that burdens us daily. When I look back on it today, I know that it was only Divine intervention that saved me.

I was forced to enter a drug rehab that was developed on the principles of a 12-Step program.

There was resistance in the beginning. I could not lower my thinking to believe I was, in fact, an addict. Hell, I was college educated, had employment skills, was from a good and respected family, not raised in the projects, smart, dressed nice, ate at restaurants, etc.

Still, in reality, I was an addict.

Once I was able to embrace that very truth was when I could finally see the light. It wasn't until I was able to address my own emotions that I was then able and ready to create noise—a noise that now rings out loudly. And, I am thankful that although forced into rehab, I received what I needed to catapult me to my next level.

December 14th of this year, I will be celebrating 18 years clean from both drugs and alcohol. Today, when people invite me out for a drink, ask me do I drink or get high, I proudly respond with, *"Naw man, haven't touched the stuff in years... I'm good."* Being the person I am, and my life, it was difficult to share this fall from grace. This was not the life I had planned. Yet, from it, has come my life's mission and purpose: to assist and guide others on a journey of redemption.

"Why me?" you ask.

Me, because I now believe I had to go through what I went through to get to where I am today — living my best life. I'm no longer ashamed because I'm finally back to "my come up."

But getting here was not easy!

"...and then I will swallow the words again wishing
for the thousandth time that you could read my mind?"
~ Celtic poetry

It is my hope that as a result of my story, along with the increasing number of highly admired celebrities who have braved the depths of self-awareness and mental health respite, other black men will become enabled to find the same courage to look within and find the clarity, peace, and fulfillment that is waiting for them.

Although it may seem as if resources are slim, there are a number of avenues one can pursue: to include, **The National Alliance on Mental Illness** (NAMI), **The Association of Black Psychologists**, **Black Mental Health Therapists** and **Black Therapist Rock** (Facebook), **Psychology Today**, and a new resource now on Twitter called **@manyougood**—a platform for men to express themselves, thoughts, emotions, and fears without judgement—just to name a few.

If you could read my mind right now, you would know that I'm hoping you will take *that leap, JUMP, just scream out HELP! I'M DYING INSIDE!* I promise you, someone will listen and guide you with passion and unconditional love.

PHYSICIAN HEAL THY SELF:
Using Non-Traditional Medicine
to Heal the Healer
By Paula S. Langford, DMin, LICSW

"You cannot dispel demons,
that you don't name."
-Dr. Paula

My life has been anything but normal.

I came into this world fighting for my life, and I have never stopped fighting. I feel there is a greater calling on my life to make this world better than I found it and help people find ways of living in this world without relying solely on traditional medicine or people who will one day fail them.

After all, we are all flawed in many ways and at times bound by the demons that have crept in or been invited within the essence of our souls. None of us, even clinicians, came into this profession unscarred. No, we have neatly, and at times not so neatly, tucked away those deep, dark secrets.

While we train, minister, and even help others to recognize their "stuff," our cellular memory continues to vibrate as if we are experiencing the very trauma we ask our clients to expose. Failing to address our trauma, causes the nastiness in the dregs of our minds, souls, and bodies to spew over to our relationships; both intimate and professional. Trauma doesn't leave the wounded healer. As good clinicians, we need to learn to recognize when our stuff is bubbling up ready to erupt.

I consider myself a Light worker who, like the reader, has experienced traumatic life events; nevertheless, every experience allows me to bring hope and healing to myself and others. Knowing what I now know, it is my desire to teach what Spirit has directed me to use in my own journey towards healing and wholeness. While others like me and the other clinicians, who write their stories in this anthology, strive to free ourselves from the addictions and traumatic experiences that we have encountered, both personally and vicariously, I want you the reader to consider, one question:

Who heals the healer?

While you are helping others work through their painful life events, who heals you? When neither your antidepressants or antipsychotic medications are working, to who and what can you turn?

Many people have heard portions of my life story, but this is the first time that I am memorializing it on paper. Some people know that I was born premature, weighing 3lbs, 4oz, and would not have been here to write my story if it had not been for my maternal grandmother's concoction of flour and water to coat my stomach allowing me to keep food down.

I grew up Catholic in East Baltimore, in a very close-knit community of struggling black families; oftentimes robbing Peter to pay Paul. I am an adult child of an alcoholic and a father who died as a result of the effects of a long history of drug addiction. My parents never married and separated when I was five. My father left us, causing my mother to fend for herself and her three children. Not many know that I survived sexual abuse by a family member, that I have had many losses; death of family and friends, as well as failed relationships.

They certainly know that I am single, barren, and sometimes find books and earning certificates, certifications, and degrees to console my desire to be a mother and a wife.

What may not be known, however, is how I have been able to survive the hell that I have been through mostly without medication, look this good, and still have a piece of mind to move through life. For me, it's only through the grace of God and my faith when no one else was available.

I have participated in individual and family therapy at various times in my life and believe in seeking professional help when necessary. After all, how can I ask someone to come in my office and disclose their deepest, most intimate secrets if I don't know the first thing about what it's like to be the patient? Not to mention, burying my traumas deep within, only caused me to release all my pain on others wherever I went.

My poor self-esteem caused me to "look for love" in all the wrong places, and past partners were not always in my best interest. Nevertheless, as Iyanla Vanzant says, *"I did the work."*

And I work on myself daily because there is still so much more to do. Nothing is impossible with God, which is why I am writing my story; the story of how I used non-traditional medicine in my healing journey.

As I take this moment to sit down and write this chapter, I have so much on my mind. I began to write this chapter several months ago, but life got in the way. My mom experienced multiple health challenges; several family members died very close together, causing me to support my aging father to travel out of town for the funerals. Chaos on the job with firings increased job responsibilities and working with less than cooperative coworkers vexed my mind and spirit. Not to mention, I had not fully grieved my brother, Sal's, death four years prior. I have suffered from several episodes of seasonal depression that have knocked me down.

As a result, I had writer's block and didn't think that I would complete my chapter. And, like you, I have been concerned about the person occupying the White House, who continues to wreak havoc on the nation and the world, and our loss of over fifty people due to a senseless shooting.

Although we clinicians experience vicarious trauma every day, we are often the last people to seek help. And there is help out there when we are riding in our cars, on the commuter trains to and from work, or just lying in bed staring at the ceiling - hoping for a peaceful night's sleep.

My mentor calls me the human ambulance. This time, in the midst of writing this chapter, I am assisting a faith-based organization with restructuring their program for community development, and I've enrolled in yet another training.

Yeah, it's a lot; and that's not all.

Trust me, I am no stranger to being busy and inundated with projects. Many times, I use my work to avoid addressing life stressors that impact my ability to be an effective community leader, daughter, church member, instructor, or friend, and it all takes a toll on my mind, body, spirit, and soul. All of these "wonderful" life lessons are happening in this season. While I look good on the outside, at times I feel like I am dying on the inside. I am no different than anyone else.

Maybe, you too, avoid addressing your trauma by focusing on your clients, or maybe you're unaware of or never considered that there is "something" more to help you balance life. What I have learned no man has revealed.

And I want to share it with you.

I have always wanted to save, help, or deliver everyone from something, *anything*, that has caused harm. Since childhood, I have felt pain in my body when I see others hurting or grieving. I entered the social work profession to offer healing. In my desire to heal the black community, I am constantly looking for ways to share information with people at the margins.

There are times when pills, salves, potions, and traditional medical treatments address the physical issues but fail to address the impact of traumatic life events on the spirit and the soul. I believe mental health professionals have only scratched the surface of the healing process; like a doctor when they have not extracted all of the cancer from the body, we leave small traces of trauma in our very being that will metastasize and resurface when we least expect it. This is why I write about the amazing complementary treatment modality, Reiki.

Every chance I get, I read anything and everything about Reiki and its ability to transform lives. I am always curious about how I can incorporate Reiki and other energy modalities in my daily life or training and mentoring practice. My Caucasian colleagues know about and utilize Reiki all over the world, while African American clinicians are just now being introduced to its astonishing properties to address past traumatic life events, substance use, eating disorders, and other mental illnesses.

There are even Reiki treatments that enhance sexual pleasure with your partner; while I won't be addressing that here, it's certainly a topic for another day. What I will tell you, is that the couples at my church, who participated in a Reiki heart connection and healing exercise, marveled at the abundant feeling of love they had for their spouses.

We've only scratched the surface of what life without traditional medicine to manage life stressors could be like. I believe that Reiki found me, and I am grateful for what I have learned in my healing process and work with others seeking relief from depression, physical pain, and despair. You don't have to believe me, find a Reiki practitioner, and try Reiki for yourself.

Journey with me as I share my story with you; a story that I believe is a gift from God that continues to assist me in the midnight hour, knowing that joy will come in the morning.

Remember, in Matthew 26: 11, Jesus said, "the poor you will always have with you." He wasn't only referring to people's finances. He also meant those who were poor in spirit and those whose hearts and souls longed for peace in mind, body, and spirit.

God has strategically placed me with some of the most wonderful enlightened teachers I've needed to train in the art of energy work with Reiki, and to learn others such as Mudras, guided meditation, EFT, and Ho'oponopono.

I'm learning even more than I could have ever imagined.

I can't tell my entire life story, but there are some miraculous times that are sure to bless your soul. "Why," you ask? Because in my faith walk, it's time! It's time for me to tell and it's time for you, as the reader to hear the story; my story of healing in non-traditional ways. I believe that we all have baggage that we need to unpack in order to maximize our effectiveness as clinicians and mental and behavioral health professionals.

I encountered many clinicians who believed that they have addressed their past trauma. I question this because I have seen many unaddressed mental health issues during meetings, at conferences, and via Facebook posts. This is by no means meant to be a criticism; rather, it is my observation from a spiritual and clinical perspective.

There are so many people relying on us, as clinicians, and it is also why it is imperative that we heal ourselves on a deeper level; both a spiritual and cellular level. That is why I use Reiki as a daily gift to myself. I have learned that I no longer need to ask permission to be kind to myself. Some of my Christian friends and family find Reiki outside of our religious tradition and doctrine; however, I believe that whatever spiritual entity to which you pray, wants you to be at your optimum health - physically, mentally, emotionally, and financially. Therefore, regardless of your faith tradition, I hope that while reading this chapter, you will open yourself up to the possibility that you can heal yourself.

What, you never thought it possible?

Maybe you have lost your faith in mankind's use of modern medicine and talk therapy. Whatever the situation, I encourage you to never lose faith in yourself.

I am a healer from a long line of women healers who healed hundreds that have crossed their paths. Like many women from the South, my grandmother was an excellent cook, who used food to comfort those who mourned. My mother has told me stories about her ability to foresee the future and ailing people with a simple touch. She was the one in the family who could soothe your soul, even if it added a few extra pounds to your hips.

In one way or another, we are all Light workers. Each of us has been given the necessary tools to heal and help people to see that life doesn't get easier, we just learn to manage the hand that we have been dealt.

In no way, do I advocate for you to throw away your blood pressure medication, discontinue your prayer life, or stop going to therapy. No, I ask you to integrate non-traditional modalities like Reiki introduced in this chapter in your use of traditional therapies and practices.

Buckle up, and let's start this journey.

Can Anything Good Come Out of Baltimore?

I know what Jesus must have felt when they questioned his healing power in the community. He grew up in a time and place where he was simply a carpenter's son. When he returned home, many who were unfamiliar with his work questioned his ability to cure in his hometown.

While I work in the nation's capital, I grew up in the eastern quadrant of Baltimore City and a product of Baltimore City Public and Catholic Schools. My neighborhood was typical of poor and working-class black families. We were close-knit, and every weekend we could be found scrubbing our white marble steps and cleaning the gutters. We didn't have a lot, but we had each other.

Like many black families, we held Sunday dinners, celebrated birthdays, and recognized school accomplishments and deaths at our matriarch's house. I was very different from my two brothers. Not only was I the only girl, but I was also my father's favorite and could convince my dad and others to give me what I wished.

I was an inquisitive child with a passion for reading. When I was about eight years old, a family member came to live with us. My parents had no idea that he was a pedophile, who ultimately sexually abused me. It was not until I was an adult and my father died that I told my mother. Rather, I buried my pain in food and engrossed myself in books as I had become even more isolated and an overachiever. I suffered in silence, eating excessively, and longing for the attention of my father.

Although my father visited, life was never the same. His presence lessened over the years, and my mother did the best that she could, but nothing satisfied my longing soul.

As time passed, I buried my pain in what never hurt: books. I studied constantly and found an escape in the pages of books that most children my age took no interest in. I went through elementary, junior high, and high school as an A+ student. Although I earned excellent grades, I was extremely sensitive and often tearful at the least thing and avoided being alone with my perpetrator and other men at family functions.

The demons of my past abuse caused me to feel unworthy. I was fearful of boys that weren't family, and I attended my junior and senior proms with my cousin, who was a close family friend because I didn't feel pretty enough to ask any of my male class-mates. It didn't help that I was not "experienced," sexually.

Nevertheless, I longed to feel pretty and worthy of true friend-ships. When I was twelve years old, I had gained enough weight to fit plus-sized women's clothes. I coped by sleeping for long hours, reading more, and secretly eating at all hours of the night. My brothers often shielded me from the ridicule of mean-spirited kids and my family tried their best to support me by joining fitness programs to help me lose weight.

I tipped the scale at three hundred seventy-eight pounds, and my health continued to be compromised by the excessive weight and depression. Regardless of what my mother gave me, or how much my family encouraged my continued success, the remaining pain continued to eat at my inner core.

With all that I had experienced, nothing deterred my yearning to know more about the supernatural. For me, there is something both scary, yet intriguing, in the supernatural. Even as a youth, I could see into the third dimension and feel the pain of others. I realized early on that I was different from my friends by seeing spiritual beings, both good and bad.

The more I saw, the more I longed to experience.

My ability to access the spiritual realm was not just for myself, but I finally felt I was special. I began to share my gifts with people, but they thought I was weird. As a young adult, I met a prophet from Bermuda, who told me of my unique calling to heal others—physically, spiritually, mentally, and emotionally.

She told me that my heart for God's people would open my spiritual eyes to see greater things that I had ever experienced. Initially, I didn't understand what the prophet meant. I was simply excited about what I could do: heal people with a touch, see into the future, and see spiritual beings.

While the prophet had helped me to make sense of many of the events that had occurred earlier in my life and the wonderful gift that had been bestowed, somehow, I missed the part about her telling me that I would spend most of my life alone. She told me that I would accomplish much, lose friends, and see even stranger spiritual beings that surrounded people, places, and things; however, it was not until several years later that her voice would resound in my head, and that I would experience just what she said. Even now, in the wake of the current president's call for a full military parade, I remember the journal entry from a dream I had almost ten years ago, of demons parading down Pennsylvania Avenue, in Washington, DC.

They were many and massive, yet I remained steadfast on the sidewalk. Still, due to my issues with low self-esteem, depression, and the negative reception I received from many people who I tried to help, I shut off my spiritual gifts.

Closing Up Shop!

I can understand what Jesus must have felt when they questioned his worth to the community. He had grown up in a time and place where he was simply a carpenter's son. Like Jesus, I felt insignificant in my family and community and needed to retreat. Instead of sharing my gift, I retreated within and remained silent about my ability to see past and future events.

After all, people only want to hear what is good. Remember, I heard only the good of what the Prophet had to tell me. In the same way, people shunned me when my "prophecies" weren't so good. But, what happens to you when others have to deal with emotional or spiritual warfare?

It becomes emotionally taxing to constantly carry traumatic life events in our cellular memory. Like the filthy blanket of Charlie Brown's friend, Linus, I carried my guilt and shame. No one talked about it, but they knew it was there; nevertheless, I continued to bury myself in my school work and to excel. I didn't know what else to do to, so I just continued to smile and pretend that life was normal.

Reflecting on my life, I now recognize that my spiritual gifts became stronger at some of the most troubling times. Romans 11:29 reminds us that, *"God's gifts and his call are irrevocable."* No matter how depressed I had become, I continued to see miraculous things happen in my life; receiving money from miraculous resources and excelling far beyond my educational level and human capacity.

This included my telling random strangers how to deal with tickets exceeding two thousand dollars while standing in the DMV line, or the time I told my soror that she would enroll in a doctoral program when I had no idea she had been applying to doctoral programs.

My spiritual connection made me the perfect vessel for my complementary and alternative modalities to work through therapeutic settings. Just think, thus far, I hadn't been introduced to

Reiki. When I thought my life would become simpler, it didn't. It only became more complicated.

A Prophet Is Not Valued In His Own Home?

What happens when you want to help, but you aren't accepted by those who have watched you stumble through life and still hold your past against you? People have long memories when someone announces their calling to a healing vocation.

I call it my vocation because this is who I now know that I am and what I was placed on this plane to do. Because of my unique calling to help others get through difficult times, grieve family losses, determine what schools to attend, address mental and physical health challenges, I had begun to be sought by people about what road they should take in their lives. I could easily tell someone how to build a business or what to say in any situation.

What about my own healing? I had earned two master's degrees each in eighteen months and a doctorate in about the same time. I accomplished all of this while single, barren, depressed and broken. As others were moving forward in addressing their "issues," I remained the wounded healer.

I steadily gained weight, suffered from low self-esteem, and smiled through my tears. That all changed during a social work training in 2006.

How Reiki Found Me!

In 2006, while attending social work training in Washington, DC, the wonderful technique of Reiki found me; ready for a change in my circumstances. Every Reiki healer will say that Reiki finds you at the time you need it most. As I have worked with energy healing modalities, I believe that all complementary healing treatments have found me that way.

The Hawaiian forgiveness modality, Ho'oponopono found me while attending a Reiki share with my cohort of Reiki practitioners. While suffering from insomnia, the Indian Mudras showed up on my Pinterest interest feed and has been with me ever since. I now incorporate them all in some form or fashion in my daily practice.

It's amazing how things happen in my life.

I've already shared with you my past sexual abuse, bouts of low self-esteem and depression, and my continued weight gain. Things seemingly couldn't get any worse except they did. I was working as a social worker in the D.C. government, and I was starting to feel like there was something more for me to do. I had started my private practice several years earlier, but business wasn't booming as they say, after my mother's contracts with Baltimore City had ended. I wanted more, but I didn't know what that more consisted of, and although I continued to feed my depression with food, I was no longer satisfied.

I had experienced one failed relationship after another and viable partners seemed to slip my grasp. I looked good on the outside, smiling and attending social events, but I felt empty and longed for a relationship.

Although I got up every day to go to work, I returned to my townhome in Baltimore, shut the door, ate until it was time to go to bed, and then cried myself to sleep.

While I had earned degrees, certificates, and certifications and was what other's saw as successful in my career, I struggled to fight back my tears daily, and nothing seemed to work to heal my hurt. I was active in my church and volunteered in my community. I taught graduate classes at the local university and helped to take care of family and friends.

In my mind, I was not successful because I had not obtained my dream of finding the right husband or bearing children. I had not earned millions of dollars nor was I the famous healer or ordained female priest that I had wanted to become. I was becoming an angry, barren woman, who continued to look for approval from others and ate my sorrows in fast food while locked away in my basement.

But, as Spirit would have it, while attending an ethics workshop, my coworker, Reverend Norma Taylor, introduced me to the wonderful healing of Reiki as she gently rested her hands on my girlfriend, Ressie, who was pregnant and having difficulty breathing.

I was curious and asked Norma, *"What did you do?"*

Even as a black Catholic, I was no stranger to the laying on of hands and something stirred in my spirit that day. Norma simply told me that she had performed Reiki on Ressie before walking away.

That incident with Ressie occurred on a Friday afternoon during our lunch break. I spent the remainder of the workshop thinking about what I had witnessed and my weekend researching, dreaming about, and contemplating this thing called Reiki. I couldn't stop thinking about what I saw Norma perform.

I was being drawn to know more.

The following Monday, I anxiously waited for Norma to arrive to work and I asked her about Reiki and how I could learn it. While in her office, Norma gave me a basic understanding of Reiki. It was at that moment that I believe my desire to heal others had reemerged in a new way. I had been a clinical therapist and was somewhat good at it. I was a good listener and, as I said earlier, I believed in the power that comes from talk therapy and traditional medicine.

Being introduced to Reiki created a stir in my soul that traditional therapists had not touched before. I had no idea the impact that Reiki and the "Reiki energy" would have in transforming my life.

What is Reiki?

When I introduce the idea of Reiki, many African Americans particularly are at a loss. The black community has either never heard of Reiki or is afraid that using integrative modalities contradicts their religious beliefs, and particularly those of the Christian faith. That's what I love about Reiki. It can be used by anyone! Reiki defined as life force (rei), and energy (ki) is the gentile energy that flows through everything. Reiki was "discovered" by Sensei (teacher) Mikao Usui, a medical doctor, in Japan while he was on a retreat in the mountains.

Like my experience, I believe that Reiki found Sensei Usui. What we know, is that when Usui was led to place his hands on various areas of his patient's body, the individual felt at ease and began to experience physical healings without medication and surgery. Usui taught Reiki classes in Japan and developed a clinic that grew in popularity.

Reiki was introduced to the West by, Hawayo Takata, Hawaiian woman of Japanese descent who had traveled to Japan. Reiki is passed down through an oral tradition from the teacher to the student and through the process called attunement (Hilton). Reiki consists of four levels; I, II, Advanced Reiki Training (ART), and Master level.

As the student is attuned to each level, the energy becomes stronger. Reiki II and higher practitioners can perform what is called distance Reiki. Distance Reiki is the ability of the practitioner to transcend time and space, healing past and future life events and individuals who are not in close proximity to the Reiki practitioner.

As amazing as it sounds, Reiki is not manipulated by the practitioner but goes where Reiki is needed for the highest good of the individual or situation.

It is through Reiki that practitioners learn to balance themselves on an emotional, spiritual, and even cellular level to promote physical, mental, and emotional healing either through touch or thought. Again, Reiki transcends time and space and is not associated with any religion.

Anyone and everyone can learn to use Reiki in their daily lives. As I learned more about Reiki, I learned that Reiki was used to treat addictions, accidents, and physical ailments. Its calming effect has been used to reduce test anxiety, treat insomnia, release blocked memories and expand spiritual awareness. In January 2008, the National Institute on Health (NIH) established the National Center for *Complementary* and *Integrative Health*, NCCIH, to study non-traditional modalities' and its impact on physical health and wellbeing.

According to NIH, "there is evidence to suggest that Reiki therapy may be effective for pain and anxiety." (2014)

After taking my first Reiki class, I knew that self-Reiki treatments would become a daily part of my life. I experienced my first Reiki class in the beautiful mountains of West Virginia with Sensei Ivy Hilton. I practiced Reiki daily and meditated on the visions and dreams that drifted into my mind. Two years later, I met and trained under my two Reiki Senseis, Faye and Joyce. For the next three years, I spent my time learning and practicing Reiki daily.

I used Reiki to complete my assignments at work and every night to balance my spiritual and emotional center. I slept better and began feeling better. I became a Reiki Master/ Teacher to train others in this new healing modality that I was showing positive outcomes for my own well-being.

As I studied the Art of Reiki and developed a stronger spiritual connection with the energy, I desired all the more to teach others to integrate Reiki in their lives to address imbalance, poor self-esteem, and trauma.

I had practiced Reiki address my self-esteem and depression. In 2007, I became aware of my continued health challenges. My weight still exceeded 300lbs, my ankles and knees hurt, and my doctor contemplated prescribing insulin as I had been diagnosed borderline diabetic.

Beyond frightened, I was angry. I longed to feel better and change my physical appearance. I had spent a tremendous amount of money and most of my life wearing plus-size clothes to hide my body. I had become weary of the excessive weight and took to a daily Reiki practice as I prepared to undergo gastric bypass surgery. I followed all of my doctor's orders: improved eating habits and exercised.

At times, I exercised seven days a week, and I loved it. Unlike my past weight loss trials, I added Reiki before, during, and after every exercise session. Although I was not losing a tremendous amount of weight, I felt more energized and focused on my physical health. Once I scheduled my surgery, I performed distance Reiki. I placed a golden white energetic light on everything from the surgeon to the instruments that would be used. The surgery went well, and I experienced no more pain than the discomfort similar to completing 100 stomach crunches. I continued my Reiki treatments until my post-op evaluation. I was given a clean bill of health and had been my physician's model patient, healing in record time.

Since my surgery, I completed my Reiki Master training and became the first Reiki Master/Teacher of the Healing Touch Reiki group of Bethesda, Maryland. I continue to use Reiki for everything, both personal and professional. My Reiki practice has been used to support healing of headaches, nausea, insomnia, and fear. In my social work practice, I have sent the loving energy of Reiki to each of the children, youth, and families on my caseload.

I observed, that with the introduction of Reiki, children and youth returned from residential treatment, achieving permanency and improving in their therapeutic programs. Even my supervisor remarked of my success in the reduction of my caseload and the improvement in the emotional regulation of older youth who had previously experienced multiple placements; moving from foster home to foster home without any life-long connections and skills that would allow them to be model citizens.

He Maketh Me To Lie Down In Peace.

Wouldn't it be wonderful if we could schedule our trials?

What if we could decide on the tremulous life events? I'm sure the world would be overpopulated because we would probably never schedule death. I would certainly not have scheduled my grandmothers' and grandfathers' transition from the physical realm. Without a doubt, I would not have asked for my brother, Salvador's, untimely death.

For two years after the dreadful day of receiving the call from my mother, informing me that a friend had found my brother dead in his East Baltimore home, I suffered from severe insomnia. Sal and I were Irish twins, being only ten months apart and inseparable as kids. He protected me when other children teased me because of my weight and fought my battles. He attended all of my graduations, and there have been many. He sat as I preached my first sermon, and he even attended the funeral service for my pet fish, Nemo. Although I couldn't convince him to stay for the repast, he took a plate of food home, shaking his head in disbelief that a grown woman couldn't flush a dead Beta fish down the toilet.

In 2016, I entered individual therapy with an excellent black female therapist to address my anger about my brother's inability to come to me for help. When I wasn't in therapy, I continuously showered myself with self-Reiki treatments throughout the day. I used Reiki prayer over my meals and began meditational walking to and from work.

At night, I performed what is called a Reiki balancing treatment, which balanced my seven chakras that run the meridian of the body from the crown of the head to just below the navel. When balancing each chakra while lying on my bed, I slow my breathing and place my hands on two chakras for a few minutes until I feel that I have applied enough Reiki energy.

Remember, Reiki goes where it is needed most.

In March 2017, I began incorporating scripture and prayer into my Reiki sessions; calling this method, Sacred Text Healing™. It is a meditation that combines Eastern integrative treatments with scared text affirmations of any religious tradition.

Each night before going to bed, I begin my Reiki treatment acknowledging my highest spiritual power! I have witnessed a profound spiritual shift in my relationship with God, from servanthood to that of an intimate relationship as the daughter, who was created in perfect love, forgiven, and capable of achieving my goals. Moving to a higher level of enlightenment and developing a stronger sense of self-worth, I recognized that my mental, emotional, and spiritual healing doesn't always generate from outside sources. Rather, I have been given the ability and permission to heal myself.

Again, this does not by any means attempt to discredit or devalue the use of mental health professionals.

However, what happens when people are not available to accept your phone call or schedule an office visit? We all must become aware that everything we need has been provided; we simply must search inwardly for the healing energy.

For me, that is Reiki.

Asante Sana (Thank you)

WITH A LOSS COMES A BIRTH
By Lennie J. Carter, MS

Beep... Beep... Beep...

This was the sound I heard every day for two weeks at Brookdale University Hospital and Medical Center in Brownsville, Brooklyn, NY. I had no idea the sound of a heart monitor would stay with me forever.

On May 1, 2008, my mother, Barbara Carter, had an accident on her way home from work. Falling on the train platform and hitting her head immediately sent her into unconsciousness.

Receiving a phone call that my mother was being admitted to the same hospital that both my paternal grandmother and great-grandmother had passed away in was not comforting. I had no idea what to expect for the recovery of my 53-year-old mother.

Was this the start of the process of no longer having my mother in my life, or was this another opportunity for my mother to show her strength by overcoming any challenge life threw her way?

Fortunately, I was in Brooklyn at my mother's apartment when I received the call that she was headed to the hospital.

Hanging up the phone, I left the apartment as fast as I could, running down seven flights of stairs.

Once I was in my car, I was determined to get an update before any medical decisions were made. So, I drove through stop signs and red lights to potentially save my mother's life, in my mind. As I walked into the emergency room, I was overwhelmed by the number of heart monitors I heard.

Beep... Beep... Beep...

Beep... Beep... Beep...

Is my mother located at one of these twenty-plus beds here in the ER? After finally getting some assistance, I was told that the ambulance hadn't arrived yet. Brookdale is known for being one of the worst hospitals in all of New York City. But, after attempting to get her taken to a better hospital, I had to settle for the fact that any head or chest injuries had to be transported to the nearest hospital.

After the ambulance had arrived, I was asked questions I never was prepared to answer.

Does your mother have any allergies?
What medications is she currently on?
Are there any health issues I should make them aware of?

I had never discussed such topics with my mother, and for the first time in my life, I couldn't ask her for an answer. As I took time to step outside and share with the rest of my family members the limited information I had, I kept reminding myself that I had to share the news positively. My energy about the circumstances would only project to others and scaring them was the last thing I wanted to do.

After debriefing my family, I stepped back into the emergency room to check the status of any tests they had conducted on my mother. The physician's assistant quickly pointed to a CAT scan of my mother's head to show where pockets of blood were forming. While trying to understand how to manage my emotions, I also had the responsibility of functioning as the messenger of information. My first phone call was to my sister in Tennessee. Giving her a status update was the toughest phone call I had to make in all of my life, but I can't remember the details of the call because it was filled with so much emotion as we tried to grasp what was going on.

Next, my aunt arrived at the hospital, which led to another emotional conversation–and probably one of the key moments that helped our relationship grow into something special. At this point, we had to come together as a family to understand how we would help my mother through this tough time.

My sister was on the first plane from Tennessee to New York the next day. The plan was for me to pick her up from the airport and head to the hospital to get a better understanding of our next steps. On a gloomy Friday, after picking my sister up from the airport, I received a call from the hospital as we were headed there.

The conversation went something like this:

"*Hello.*"
May I speak to Lennie Carter?
"*Yes, this is he. Is everything okay with my mother?*"

I'm the attending doctor, and the reason we are calling you is that your mother's brain has swelled so much we need to cut her skull open to relieve the pressure. If we don't do it, she will not survive the swelling.

"Do the surgery!"

I had to have this conversation while driving on the Jackie Robinson Parkway, a curvy highway that was built through a cemetery. Although the conversation made me feel anxious about needing more time, I understood I had to stay focused on my driving if I was going to get to the hospital and be of any use to my mother. Shortly afterward, my sister and I arrived at the hospital and waited a few hours until the surgery was complete.

The next time I saw her, my mother was on a gurney with half of her head shaved with bandages wrapped around it. It hadn't even been twenty-four hours, and my life changed, literally, overnight.

Beep... Beep... Beep...

I spent the next two weeks becoming very familiar with that sound, the indicator that there was life in an unconscious body. Each day that I spent at the hospital, the more the sound caused flashbacks. Visiting my unconscious mother for two weeks straight was not good for my mental health. The flashbacks I got would have me question every step of my life, and my mother's, that got us to this point.

Beep... Beep... Beep...

The sound of beeps is a sign of life. It is a confirmation that your loved one's heart is still beating and there is anticipation that prayer, love, and hope will heal them to make it home. The first few days were the toughest. I experienced a roller coaster of emotions in the beginning. The sound of the beeps gave me comfort in knowing my mother still was in the process of healing.

Beep... Beep... Beep...

The common theme for my flashbacks was the previous family health emergencies and the loss of loved ones throughout my teenage years. The first time I remember hearing that beeping sound was when I visited my maternal grandfather in the hospital while he was receiving his chemotherapy treatments for lung cancer.

I was 15 years old when my grandfather was diagnosed with cancer. Finding out this information as a teenager in the 90s was confusing. New information about cancer was developing yearly, but there was no definitive way for me to understand as a teenager that diseases can manifest in the human body and cause numerous health concerns.

Faced with trying to understand how the man who taught me how to fish and to play spades, poker, and pokeno by the age of seven was now in a position of life and death. I had a lot of questions with no one to get answers from. Questions like *Will he make it home alive?* as I watched him get sicker with each chemotherapy treatment.

My grandfather was a World War II veteran who spent time in Okinawa. I could recall war stories he would share and learned how he navigated the world as a black man in the United States during the 1920s, 40s, and 50s. I could not fathom the idea that cancer would kill my grandfather when he had survived being robbed in our building one hot summer day while I played outside.

This was an unfamiliar place for me. To watch the man I had grown up with, who was strong and independent, face being dependent to survive, was hurtful. So, I visited my grandfather in the hospital to let him know the lessons learned wouldn't be forgotten. While I was there, all I heard was...

Beep... Beep... Beep...

My grandfather, Archie Ray, passed away on March 5th, 1996, just a month after I turned 16. I don't remember crying much after hearing the news, because I didn't know how to feel. I had previously experienced losing my Aunt Kathy and my great-grandmother, Nan, but both of these deaths happened at an age where growing up in the hood and learning that someone passed away was common.

If you have never experienced a funeral with an immediate family member, let me tell you the process as a teenager can be overwhelming. In this scenario, I had to watch my grandmother deal with losing a husband and my mother deal with losing her father. The sadness that I had over losing my grandfather wasn't shared by all my family members, though. As a child you don't realize how everyone has a different relationship with a person you look up to as a role model, but as the stories unravel you can understand that a person can leave behind darkness with death.

My grandfather drank his fair share of alcohol—enough that some may have considered him an alcoholic. I can attempt to share all the reasons why a black man who is a U.S. Army veteran from North Carolina, born in 1923 drank so much, but I'm sure you can imagine the amount of racial, mental health, and employment challenges he had throughout his life.

My grandfather's drinking exposed me to psychosis for the first time. He would drink liquor (spirits) and walk aimlessly around the house speaking to himself. And, if he drank a little too much, he would vomit. To this day, I cannot smell E&J Brandy without thinking about my grandfather and those moments of psychosis. Are all of my good times with my grandfather invalid due to his dark side that I was unaware of?

As I got older and learned more about society, I began to wonder. *Was he really the one to blame for his challenges, or were they the result of living through the Great Depression, the army draft era, and during the time that we were still segregated as a country? Was who he became a mirror image of black men in America? Did my grandfather represent the struggle?*

Beep... Beep... Beep...

A week had passed with my mother in the hospital, and there had been minimal progress in her improvement. Extended family would visit the hospital with their support, and family members who were in the healthcare industry as doctors or nurses shared how bad the situation was. As we entered into the second week of my mother's unconsciousness, the steady rhythm of her heart monitor continued to get louder and louder.

I began to internalize the feelings of losing a loved one. Day after day I was in a place where this loud beeping sound had become a part of my daily life. I was almost a slave to it. As each day passed with my mother on that dreaded machine, my mood continued to get numb.

My emotional immune system literally felt no pain. I had a responsibility as a black man to take the lead with my family. We had prayer every night and evaluated every option we could to prepare for the worst while hoping for the best.

Beep... Beep... Beep...

Were these the feelings my dad and his sisters felt when my grandmother, Lorraine Carter, suffered a heat stroke in April of 2002? I was at a point in my life that I was fighting to cross the bridge of being from the hood and becoming a statistic to having a college degree and entering corporate America. I was in my fourth year of college when my paternal grandmother suffered that stroke. With her in the hospital on life support, where would I find the strength to carry on?

Three days later, my phone rang; it was my father letting me know that my grandmother had passed away. All I remember is feeling a full-body rush of anger. I began to reflect on life, and the 22 years I had the fortune of spending with her.

Then anxiety kicked in as I thought of the effect this would have on my family; especially on her husband, my paternal grand-father, an independent man who was only one year away from his 50th anniversary, and, unfortunately, with the untimely passing of my grandmother, showed signs of depression.

I use that term very loosely because anyone who knew my grandfather knew that he was the type of man who would never categorize himself as depressed.

He didn't get depressed; he managed and moved on.

Three months later, my grandfather began to cough up blood. This was odd because he had a clean bill of health before my grandmother's passing. Following an examination and biopsy, my grandfather found out he had cancer, with masses on his lung, hip, and spine. Aggressive chemo treatment was the only solution to slowing or eliminating it.

Graduating in December of 2002 was an opportunity to bring joy to my grandfather's life, eight months after the passing of my grandmother. Unfortunately, my grandfather was too ill with his chemo treatments to attend my graduation. Although he was able to win that battle in his fight against cancer, cancer eventually won the war. My grandfather passed away in March of 2003. At the age of 23, I had to begin thinking about what my next steps would be in helping my family and those around me. Looking in the mirror, I saw a black man with every obstacle in front of him, but who was also taught by two war veterans on the real art of the Black man's war to survive the worst circumstances.

As Black men in America, we not only have to fight for our freedom and for our voice to be heard, we also have to provide for and protect our women and children. Is it possible to succeed in our country when black men are held to low standards in America, while at the same time, held to the highest standard as a leader in the community?

This is a question I ask myself every day. How can I be my best, based on the view of black males from society?

The Transition

Beep... Beep... Beep...

I woke up on May 16, 2008, with the plan I had for the last two weeks—visit my mother in the hospital and evaluate any and every approach that can be taken to give her the best opportunity to recover. I'm not sure if it was because it was a Friday, but we had a few more visitors than usual stop by the hospital that day.

There was a point in the day that is a blur because all I remember is that my lifeline did not sound the same anymore. You know what I'm talking about. Yeah, that beeping sound I mentioned that is etched in my head. Once that secure and familiar sound became a fearful sound of inconsistency I needed to take a moment to myself in the bathroom.

Staring at myself in the mirror I had a one-word question: *Why?*

My aunt came to get me from the bathroom to let me know that my sister needed me, and we were approached and quite vehemently declined to sign a "Do Not Resuscitate Order" (DNR).

We had to watch our mother flatline multiple times.

As my mother transitioned, so did I. I continued to carry that numb feeling that emerged in the second week of my mother being in the hospital, and after watching her leave my life, that numbness has been buried in me ever since. It took a major toll on my mental health and added fuel to the fire of pre-existing suicidal thoughts. I was an emotionless robot, concentrating on career success rather than my mental health success.

Business Became My Heart Monitor

Two years before my mother passed away I became a full-time entrepreneur. Starting my career in the tech startup industry led me to a world of information and my determination to learn everything I could about technology was a dream come true. There is no better learning tool than hands-on experience.

Being an entrepreneur will test your mental health on a consistent basis. Then to add the layer of losing my mother to the journey only complicated my emotional stability. After my mother passed away the business became my lifeline. I felt a sense of ownership for every failure of the business. When the business was at its lowest points, I struggled to connect with people due to the emotional damage I already suffered.

As I continued to work harder, we began to see a little bit of growth as a company, expanding our customer base and growing our staff. Then, when most people realized a recession was beginning to take a turn for the worst, I was also struggling with the sad news of my business partner being diagnosed with stage four lymphoma. This is similar to your lead pitcher or starting quarterback being injured, but this real-life example meant life or death for a partner who had become a brother.

Thankfully, a loved one referred me to therapy, and I began to see results from addressing my grieving of my mother and previous loved ones lost.

Outside of the freedom you have in therapy to be yourself, most therapists allow you to set your own goals and plans. Building a relationship with a good therapist gave me an outlet to learn the steps of the grieving process.

The Ghost of Grief

As my partner experienced his battle with cancer, I was caught up with focusing on the business and grieving at the same time. I began to learn about the five stages of grieving and the impact it can have on the processes of grieving, especially for an analytical person such as myself.

Denial

The first stage of grief is denial, and being from the hood, I've lived through denial myself as I've seen others do. But, one of the biggest things that can cause someone from the hood to be removed emotionally from death is the fact that it is a part of our everyday reality. In communities of color, the denial line can easily get blurred in a therapy session.

There is a sense of denial through picking up the phone to call the person or still hearing their voice in your head when things in life get rough. My therapist understood that the denial stage was more of a guide than a ruler to measure my denial.

Denial comes in many forms: business, relationships, and grief. I've used denial as a defense to stay in relationships longer than necessary or not changing the direction of a business as soon as I should have. Denial lives in all of us. We need to do as much as possible to understand it is part of the process and not resist the fact that we can live in denial from perspectives you may not have seen yet.

Anger

Progressively, most people transition to stage two, which is anger. Being from Brownsville, Brooklyn stage two is where we began. I was angry from the day I found out my mother was on her way to the hospital.

I had anger in me *before* I received that call, and knowing my mother was not well only added fuel to that anger.

This is a dangerous stage for communities of color. I know people who are still at this stage because the choices they made while grieving caused them to get arrested for crimes committed while grieving. I had my fair share of poor choices while in stage two, and I'm fortunate to survive the anger and fire that burned inside of me at that time.

Therapy helped me manage my anger and find ways to stay away from the triggers that get me fired up. The clarity that therapy gave me on my frustrations saved me from harming myself through some of my deepest suicidal thoughts. I've watched all of my loved ones go through the anger phase while grieving and some are still recovering from the emotional damage they experienced through it all.

Bargaining

Feeling guilty sat with me while I was still in stage two. However, my anger escalated in stage three because I felt there were chances for me to help my mother make the transition out of Brooklyn. *What if she was living in another state? Would this have happened?* was a common question I would ask myself.

Therapy guided me in understanding that "only if" could not be a theme if I planned to grow through the experience. The longer I held onto the "only ifs," the longer it would take for me to find success in other areas of my life.

Depression

The fourth stage is depression, and I promise you that I know this stage well. I believe I spent my whole life depressed and I masked it by keeping my mind busy with mental escapes. I came to realize that the biggest indicator of whether I'm depressed or not is my appetite. As greedy as I am, I tend to lose my appetite when I'm depressed.

Families in the Black communities don't necessarily believe in or support you when you're going through depression; you are viewed as being weak. This is a common theme as a black man. Had my grandfather sought help for his past experiences, maybe his drinking and pain over the years would have provided clarity for him to approach his relationship with our family differently.

I began to see that my depression was no different than anyone else's in my community. We had similar experiences, struggles, and, in some cases goals, but the trauma we experienced created an emotionally guarded environment.

There was no way you can define yourself as an individual when the world has defined you and your community before you were born. Depending on the age of your mother she was more than likely judged while pregnant with you. Going to therapy helped me unpack the emotions of depression and continued to help me manage my day-to-day feelings of grief.

Acceptance

The final stage is acceptance—getting to the point of accepting the new reality of no longer speaking to, seeing, or hearing your loved one. Removing a phone number from your contact list or going through the process of giving away their possessions takes a lot of emotional strength.

The time we have to invest in transitioning our routines that will no longer include a loved one is a process. It took a lot for me to accept the fact that my mother would never meet my children or see any other future endeavors I accomplish.

With a Loss Comes a Birth

As I continued my entrepreneur journey and my partner's cancer went into remission, I continued to use the knowledge I was learning from therapy in my everyday life. Applying these new-found mental health tools gave me the strength to continue being an effective business partner and to grow our business into a success.

Then, on May 17, 2015, my brother, Che Carter, had to come to grips with the loss of his childhood friend, Chinx. Before rapper Chinx had the respect of rap mogul Diddy and fellow artist French Montana, he was just known as Lionel Pickens from Far Rock (Far Rockaway, Queens). Far Rock was home to another slain up-and-coming rapper, Stack Bundles.

I had to deliver the crushing news the day after the seventh anniversary of my mother's death.

Again, mentally, I wasn't in the best headspace since I had to relive the passing of my mom. However, I had to be strong for my brother during this heart-wrenching moment.

Have you ever heard a grown man sob uncontrollably? It's something that will be etched in my mind forever.

Given the circumstances of Chinx's untimely death, I knew my brother needed more than familial support to get him through this tough time. This was when I realized that I needed to combine my tech knowledge with my experience as a black man struggling to find mental health resources for myself and my brother. So, I created a solution. I created a web and mobile platform that is a client engagement and referral tool for mental health professionals while providing a safe place for people of color to find mental health resources.

I wish a product like TruCircle existed back then. I would have known exactly where to send Che to get the emotional and mental support he needed. Essentially, TruCircle came about because I wanted to help my brother cope with a loss. Now, I want to help all Brothers.

As I continued with therapy, I began to understand that my previous approach to mental and emotional wellness was futile. Discussions with my therapist allowed me to understand the differences between coping and receiving professional help. I realized that listening to music—even music that expressed my pain—or sharing my struggles with my barber was not enough. Armed with this understanding, I set out to make a change in the mental health arena in underserved communities.

Through my personal challenges, I recognized that there are four key pillars to helping others get through tough times.

1. Remove the stigma

Let's remove the stigma that's associated with mental illness. Some people are too afraid to seek therapy because they have been led to believe it's a sign of weakness. Simply telling your boy to "man up" is not going to give him the solace he needs to deal with his problems. Remember, mental illness does not discriminate, and it could be anyone's reality.

2. Provide access

We need to provide more access to mental health professionals. Technology can help us bridge this gap. If we can get a dog walker on demand, then there is no reason why we cannot have access to mental health resources.

3. Mitigate cost

Getting help from a therapist is not as expensive as one might think. Not only are there insurance plans that pay for mental health services, but many city and state agencies have heavily discounted (and at times free) mental health resources available to all people.

4. Find the right information and match

People struggling with a mental health issue need a therapist with cultural competence. Finding a therapist who won't judge you based on your socioeconomic background and appearance is key.

No one wants help from someone they think will judge them. Growing up in Brownsville, Brooklyn, earning my bachelor's and master's degrees from Stony Brook University, and working out of the largest therapeutic community in New York City, will allow me to merge my life experiences with more than a decade of tech experience to change the world for the mental health of people of color.

The adage, "It takes a village to raise a child" applies to everyday life, including mental health awareness. Since a community or village is a group of people with shared values, goals and backgrounds, let me share with you what I'm doing to contribute to the four pillars of mental health awareness. I'm using technology to tackle all four pillars—judgment-free therapy, access to a therapist, affordable therapy, and the maintenance of a roster of culturally conscious therapists.

If we as a community can work toward strengthening these four pillars of mental health access, it will play a huge role in helping the Black community become more comfortable addressing their mental health issues.

The true power of TruCircle is by us providing underrepresented mental health professionals with the technology tools needed to enhance their clients' experience. Our features focus on client engagement to help providers save time and become more efficient while they grow their practices. Trucircle does this by increasing a providers' reach through our online directory.

We enhance their communication with our HIPAA compliant video conferencing for 1-on-1 and group session hosting. We also offer client management tools to make day-to-day tasks simpler.

TruCircle is the result of the pain I suffered when losing my mother and the hope I gained while going to therapy. I'm alive today because of therapy, and now I recommend therapy to everyone. Therapy is just as important as going to the dentist. If you don't go to the dentist, you can get cavities and lose your teeth; luckily there are dentures for that.

Unfortunately, your brain can't be replaced the same way your dentures can be, so going to therapy can be the difference between life and death!

----Flatline

SEX, SEXUALITY, AND GENDER:
The Unspoken Connection
To Mental Health
By Chasity Chandler, LMHC

If I told you that I was an insecure-secure, extroverted, cis-gender, heterosexual female who is a sex-positive advocate, LGBTQ+ affirming mental health & sex therapist, you would only get a glimpse of who I am.

I know that is a mouth-full, and throughout this chapter, I will explain what a lot of those terms mean, and how the work in the areas of sex, sexuality, and gender has affected myself and others I have encountered in my lifetime.

You are being addressed by the girl who was the "tomboy" and the "outcast"; just a little too loud to be considered a "young lady," a little too open and free to be considered "normal," and a little too far left and assertive to be completely accepted by her professional peers who don't look like her.

Growing up, I knew that there was something special about me. Not because that was what my parents or family told me, but because there is no way I could have gone through what I did and still be able to stand before you, the empowered, ambitious, and determined woman I am today.

My first sexual experience was with someone I trusted; someone I cared for, and someone who was supposed to protect me and show me the rights and wrongs of life. Instead, they would slip into my bed when I visited their house, touch me in ways a seven-year-old didn't know was wrong, and insert pieces of their self into my pure flesh; swearing me to secrecy.

This was not the only time this would happen, and eventually, this was something I would grow to believe was normal. I was continuously told not to talk about things that happened in our house or family, because 'the people' would come and get us. I think this *"What happens in our house, stays in our house"* mentality, coupled with my not knowing that what was happening to me was wrong, led to a path of engaging in sexual activity at an early age; allowing boys to sell me a dream and whisper sweet nothings in my ear, while enjoying parts of me in a physical way.

Soon, I began to feel that the way males showed me love was by being sexually intimate with me, fostering grave insecurities when it came to forming romantic relationships, and a sexually open-minded curiosity.

Although these—and other—horrible things happened to me, my life has always taken the path of being a helper.

People knew that they could come to me about anything, and they never feared judgment or that their business would be aired out to the masses. This, and other personal experiences of my life, will be shared as an opportunity to educate and empower you to overcome whatever you've been through, what society says about you, and how you can address it.

PART II

Some say that mental health has the greatest stigma in the African American or black community, but I'm here to share that it's not. Rather, I would argue that sex, sexuality, and gender hold the biggest amount of stigma or taboo in our culture, and inadvertently can lead to mental illness and additional harmful situations.

That is a pretty strong statement. How does one come to that conclusion? We are raised to be "straight," meet someone nice, settle down which may or may not include marriage depending on our family's beliefs, and have kids. Some of it is due to a lack of knowledge; some of it is due to the discomfort with being 100 percent open about who we are, and strong gravitation toward religion and searching for a sense of self.

Sex is a natural part of life and is a huge part of who we are as human beings. In fact, ignoring your sense of self as a sexual being, and denying yourself the opportunity to explore, can lead to other mental health implications in your romantic and interpersonal relationships with others, as well as how we parent our children.

When we're born, we are told that we are a boy or a girl. From there, we are told what it means *and looks like* to be a boy or a girl; what to wear, how to interact with others, and what is (or is not) acceptable, based on our assigned gender at birth.

We haven't even formed a personality, likes, or dislikes, our moral fibers still being developed; yet, people, those closest to us, and those who are responsible to show us how to love, put limitations and boundaries on what we can be, what we can look like, and how we can express ourselves.

Those who have been through sexual abuse are still sexual beings. Those who are unsure of their sexuality, or don't subscribe to the heteronormative values placed on our society today, still deserve to be loved and to experience love.

Those who do not fit the cookie cutter views of gender, as it relates to male and female, are still human beings and deserve to be treated as such.

This isn't an "us" versus this thing, or a right or wrong thing. It is a healthy versus unhealthy thing. Neither I, nor others, deserved the things that we have been through, but we do deserve to be the healthy sexual beings we were meant to be. I'm saying that to say this...

Your sexual health and mental health
is just as important as your physical health.

So, someone says "Why would you want to write about sex?" "People don't talk about sex." "That is a private subject." Yes, sex has traditionally been a very private subject; virtually undiscussed and seems to have plenty of public ramifications in today's society.

However, not talking about it doesn't stop people from doing it, and having incorrect information only puts themselves and others at risk.

Sex is not taboo, nor is it dirty.

We are born into this world as sexual beings. Why not talk about it? What could it hurt?

Many times, those in the African American/Black community are exposed to sex at a very early age; more often than not, without consent. Incest and molestation tend to be a topic that is less talked about, but extremely prevalent in our society. Could it be that speaking to our children about age-appropriate sexual topics helps to prevent this?

If our parents and grandparents had told us something about sex that was more than "don't do it," "you're gonna get pregnant," "sex is only for marriage," or not discuss it at all, would this have protected our innocence a little longer?

Speaking openly about sex with our youth is also something most see as taboo. I was recently asked to write in an online magazine for parents on the subject of *how to talk to your kids about sex*. The preceding topic was on abstinence. Here is a little snippet of what I shared:

"Abstinence is the information our children receive in school-sponsored sex education classes now. They are taught to abstain from having sex because it will lead to pregnancy and sexually transmitted infections (STI's). The truth is sex can lead to STI's and pregnancy, but there are more aspects to sex than those two topics.

I think it is important for everyone to understand that as human beings we're sexual beings and there is a need to become educated on what that truly means starting with ourselves. As parents most, not all, weren't allowed to talk about sex because our parents were not comfortable with the subject, it went against their religious principles, or they lacked the ability and information to help us become sexually healthy, informed individuals. This sometimes contributes to a peak in sexual curiosity, experimentation, rebellion and more."

No one is saying that your "birds and bees" talk has to be explicit; just simply saying that age-appropriate conversations need to start as early as two or three. This could begin with using proper terminology of genitalia, like penis and vagina, and avoiding nicknames for these body parts.

The habit of using "pet names" or "nicknames" for genitalia can contribute to our children's inability to communicate if there is inappropriate touching, or other acts, as it relates to them sexually.

I know we always think of things being really innocent and that we don't need to worry about that with our children because we are extra-attentive; however, don't let our children spend the night over at people's houses that we don't know, with the hope that they will be able to tell us.

The reality of the situation is that most people affected by childhood sexual abuse are violated by someone they know. It is not the strangers that we have to worry about so much (not saying that they aren't a threat at all), but it's the pastors, teachers, coaches, family friends, and even family members.

It can be hard to believe that those we love and trust the most are oftentimes the very ones who cause us harm.

To be clear, sexuality is simply the way we express ourselves as sexual beings and how we experience being sexual. This is not to be confused with one's sexual orientation, which is who you are attracted to emotionally, physically, sexually, and spiritually. A person's sexuality can be fluid and non-specific. It is such a huge part of who we are and how we show up in the world. The ability to be authentic in this area is even more important, but many individuals are not able to do that for fear of judgment, ridicule, or their own beliefs surrounding their sexuality itself.

This is an arena I know all too well specializing in LGBTQ+ community. Many of my clients come to me after not knowing where to turn to get help and assistance, being ostracized by their families and feeling isolated and alone due to them "being different" or "not being straight." This heteronormative rhetoric is huge in the black community for sure. Being black and gay or trans comes with even more barriers and challenges than those who are non-black.

Society has their views, biases, and opinions of the LGBTQ+ population, and so does the black community. Most of which are rooted out of religious beliefs and personal preferences. To be gay, trans, non-binary, etc., in the black community is to be judged, ridiculed, and more in some cases even by those that you are seeking help from.

There have been a lot of discussions in several therapy communities on social media regarding sex, sexuality, and gender and let's just say that these are still topics that can't be had in a mature and professional manner with black and brown helpers.

Most of the discussions end up in arguments and being shut down by the administrators due to personal bias, lack of research-based responses, and A LOT of assumptions that are passed on as fact. This is those professionals "junk," and needs to be addressed in supervision, consultation, and possibly more. There is work to be done on how empathetic we can be to those who come to us for help and to know when to refer to a more qualified professional when our experience, expertise, and possibly personal biases would not be sufficient to assist those seeking help.

The fact of the matter is that LGBTQ+ folk exist in our communities and they deserve to receive quality care as everyone else.

PART III

I have touched on the importance of open and honest discussions when it comes to discussing sex, sexuality, and gender. Starting early has the greatest impact. Seeking professional help from a qualified professional can make a huge difference in your mental health and sexual health.

Yes, I went to therapy. I needed to work on my own stuff and prepare myself for the work that I was about to do as a therapist. I knew that working in the substance abuse field and me pursuing my dream of becoming a sex therapist would require me to be in a healthy space when it came to topics related to sex. Opening up to those close to me about the sexual abuse that I endured as a child was not an easy thing, but it was so necessary.

I was at the end of my master's program and asked for suggestions from a trauma therapist from my professors. They directed me to a trained traumatologist who fully explained EMDR (Eye Movement Desensitization and Reprocessing) to me. This entire process required me to be vulnerable and transparent.

He suggested this modality of therapy as he had over thirty years' experience in this realm and felt that this would be the best course of action.

Five to six sessions was all it took.

The beauty of this process was I didn't have to go into detail about what happened to me. The rounds of processing could take place with just me thinking about the details and telling him how I was being affected by the reprocessing. No more nightmares, flashbacks, intrusive thoughts, etc.! I was free of the vivid memories of my innocents being stolen in my childhood.

This also gave me my power back. I was no longer a victim; I became a survivor. More than ten years later and I am still helping those who are dealing with sexual violence and attaining relief of those symptoms with EMDR and other therapy methods.

This also helped me be able to gain more control over the sexual situations that I allow myself to get involved in. No longer seeking this sense of false approval, acceptance, and love from men through sex, but having the ability to make healthy sexual decisions that result in better mental health for me. Understanding that consent is mine to give and take away, and I have the right to do so without feeling guilty or obligated to engage in sex when I do not want to, regardless of who the interaction is with.

Coming to terms with what happened to me helped me embrace who I am. That woman that I described at the beginning of this section that continues to work towards being unapologetically me. Embracing my strengths and exploring my weaknesses in a way that allows for improvement while granting myself grace. Taking my personal experiences and professional growth in a direction to help and assist others has been a huge part of my healing.

To know that I am able to help others who have been through similar things and prevent this from reoccurring. This has not only helped me to be more comfortable about talking with others about my abuse but also helped me to do more as a parent to better equip my children to have the words and knowledge necessary to ask for help. I was always able to speak about sex in a general manner and even did in-home adult sex parties.

Heck, I still do.

My passion for helping others feel open, safe, and affirming in their sexual experiences has been some of my best work in and outside of my office.

When a client can call my practice and feel comfortable to be open about the issues and concerns that they have because we are inclusive in our language, open about our role in creating and holding a safe space for them to freely explore their sex, sexuality, and gender it warms my heart.

Hearing the shame and fear that is deeply rooted in receiving help for sexual issues for fear of judgment and not knowing how the professional would respond.

A person who is within the LGBTQ+ spends about 50 percent of their mental energy on staying safe. Yes, I said staying safe. I know we are in 2018 and most think that everyone is generally safe and there is no need for extra precautions, but the reality is that is not the case. In many states, a person can still lose their job and apartment for being LGBTQ+, and there are no real repercussions that will occur.

Could you imagine being able to be fired because of who you love and are sexually involved with? Would you be open and honest about who you are at your core if you knew it would be met with scrutiny, oppression, and prejudice?

Most of us wouldn't.

However, these are some of the issues my clients have to focus on in their daily interactions with others. A lot of these concerns come as a result of their interactions with other helping professionals as well. We take a vow to first do no harm, but when we are not aware of our own biases and how they can impact the therapeutic process we can cause more harm than good.

I am determined to help other professionals learn how to create a sex-positive environment and to aid in the ability to provide safe, affirming, and inclusive services to all. It is necessary for the clients that we serve to get quality services as what we do is not just talk. As Deran Young, founder of **Black Therapists Rock,** always says, *"We are working with people's brains."*

So, let's make sure we are doing our part with staying on top of our continued education and additional training and services so that we are not adding to the stigma of our profession, but truly doing the work to make a difference.

The purpose of this chapter is to have you think about your attitude around sex. Did you have "the talk" about sex when you were growing up? What were the messages you received when it came to sex? Were your parents open, or was it like crickets whenever you asked? How does one determine what is or is not acceptable sexually?

Those messages and attitudes that are modeled to us can shape how we view sex in our adult lives and future relationships. I see this a lot in my work with couples. The relationship dynamics that are modeled from our parents, or the couples that we were connected to, really define how we feel relationships should be; whether they show affection to one another, the phrase *"I love you"* is used, constantly argued or fought, or if they never spent quality time together.

Intimacy and communication are huge parts of this as well. One might ask what does intimacy consist of, how does it show up in a relationship, and how do you keep it there?

A definition of intimacy that was given in my textbook said that intimacy is the ability to experience an open, supportive, tender relationship with another person without fear of losing one's own identity in the process. A barrier that I see with a lot of the couples and individuals I work with is that they cannot connect intimately due to a lack of communication. If you can learn how to communicate effectively, most problematic areas in a relationship can be improved. Having the ability to open up about how you feel and what you need, can be a complete game changer; not to mention, it will cut down on conflict and arguments.

One tends to feel closer and more connected when they feel understood and heard.

This could increase intimacy, desire, and ultimately make significant changes in your sex life. These aspects of our beliefs, views, and assumptions of sex, affection, and love play a major role in our ability to model such behavior in our own lives. It's far past the time of allowing incest, molestation, and sex-talk taboos to keep us from being who we were destined to be as people. Together, we can make a difference.

This chapter - *and this book* - is just the start.

ABOUT THE AUTHORS

Growing up with an incarcerated father and a mother who struggled with mental illness and substance abuse, **Deran Young** gained knowledge and experience of discrimination, poverty, and social services at a very early age. It was no shock that she later decided to pursue a career as a helping professional.

After obtaining her Bachelor's degree in Social Psychology, Deran moved to pursue a Master's in Public Administration and a Master's in Social Work. While obtaining her Masters in Social Work at the University of Texas, she was blessed with an amazing opportunity to visit Ghana, West Africa twice, first as a graduate assistant and then during a final field placement/internship.

During her six-month stay in Ghana, Deran created a Guidance & Counseling Center at a High School in a neighborhood that has been historically identified as a population of lower socio-economic status. During her work there, she also created a scholarship program titled "Choices" and conducted a cultural identity field trip for students to learn about African and African American History firsthand. Her passion for culture and diversity lead her to further explore issues of social justice and social psychology.

Deran's current areas of expertise include International Social Work, Gender Issues, and Trauma/Anxiety Disorders.

Tiffany L. Reddick is a licensed professional counselor and therapeutic lifestyle change coach specializing in millennial mental health. She helps purpose, performance, and profit-driven professionals develop and implement wellness strategies that allow them to love their best life while changing the world and collecting their coins!

After gaining ten years of experience in the human services field, a life coach certification, and an obscene amount of student loan debt, she was faced with the realization she was in an unhealthy relationship with the career she once adored. She launched SavvyLife Group in hopes of reclaiming her schedule and her sanity while empowering others to do the same by engaging in the work they love effectively and sustainably.

Tiffany believes in mindfulness, trap music, and her ability to change the world and make it to happy hour on time. Due to her work as a traveling counselor, she is hardly home, but always reppin' [Metro] Atlanta, Georgia.

To learn more about Tiffany or inquire about working with her, visit savvylifegroup.com or email Hello@Savvylifegroup.com. She can also be found lurking on the gram under the handle @SavvyLifeTip.

Khalilah Williams is a Marriage and Family Therapist who works with her clients on exploring and identifying their areas of strengths and resilience. She has supported individuals, couples and families as they identify and address problematic patterns in their lives and relationships.

Through her own experience and working with mothers, Khalilah founded the organization "Mommy Take off Your Cape", which promotes self-care and psycho-education to mothers. She is also the host of an internet radio show titled "Mommy Take off Your Cape" featured on Beacon of Light Radio, with the goal being to empower women to care for themselves without guilt or shame, to increase their self-esteem, and to provide them with more effective parenting skills and strategies on how to balance the different roles they have more efficiently.

Khalilah supports women and their families as they address maternal mental health and the internal dialog women experience after giving birth.

Chautè Thompson, LMHC is a licensed clinician, speaker, author, consultant, educator, transformation coach and certified family mediator. Ms. Thompson offers life-changing strategies, empowerment, personal development, mental and emotional health messages to schools, churches, conferences, workshops, and seminars. She is passionate about helping others GROW mentally, emotionally and spiritually into the best version of themselves.

Ms. Thompson is the owner of Inspiring Hope Counseling Service, LLC (IHCS) a private practice in Florida. IHCS focuses on helping families strengthen their family unit helping ALL families become healthier and happier. IHCS also specializes in women's issues, transitions, parenting support, anger management, anxiety depression and PTSD. Christian Counseling is available, in addition to counseling for the deaf and hard of hearing.

Ms. Thompson is the founder of Brand New Me, LLC (BNM). BNM focuses on providing resources, education, and empowerment enabling women to rediscover and redefine themselves GROWING past the pain of divorce and life-changing events, adjusting to numerous transitions, becoming whole and living happier/healthier lives.

To learn more or contact Ms. Thompson:

www.inspirehopehealthhealing.com
www.chautethompson.com
info@chautethompson.com

Phoenixx Love, LCSW is a Holistic Therapist, Wellness Consultant, Educator, and Author. She is the Owner of Healer's Haven Holistic Health and Wellness Consulting Services. Phoenixx has over 20 years of Administrative and Clinical experience in Integrated Healthcare, behavioral science, clinical psychology, child welfare and the healing arts. Phoenixx is currently an Adjunct Professor and Advisor at Hunter College in Manhattan, New York. Formerly, she was a Mental Health Administrator and Professional Development Trainer for the NYS Office of Mental Health.

Healer's Haven is a sanctuary. As a Certified Ra Sekhi Reiki and Vibrational Sound Healing practitioner, Phoenixx specializes in synchronizing psychotherapy, holistic healing, spiritual practices and evidence-based interventions to help her clients manage stress, reduce symptoms and maladaptive behavior. Phoenixx offers customized training, EAP services, and workshops to help businesses and organizations achieve their wellness and productivity goals.

Phoenixx Love is the author of *If I Should Die Before I Wake: Your Journey to Awakening Your Calling*. A healing tool and solution-focused guide that consists of 50 transformative messages designed to enlighten and inspire people to discover their life purpose.

She is also an ambassador for Mental Health Awareness; Healing from a Holistic perspective.

Reveal. Heal. Live On Purpose.

To learn more, visit: www.ahealershaven.com

Nicole Thompson is a Certified School Psychologist. For the past five years, she has worked as a Psychologist in a large urban high school. Her role has been to collaborate with the students, their families, the staff, and other stakeholders from the school and community to better serve the student population.

She is a mentor and founder of a female empowerment group named Frankford's Finest Females which sparked the creation of an annual all-female Black history program.

Also known as The Urban School Psychologist, Nicole is the founder of Reverse the Adverse, a trauma-competent training program. Her mission is to raise awareness and teach educators how to better serve urban students plagued with trauma.

Nicole completed her graduate studies at Philadelphia College of Osteopathic Medicine, and her undergraduate studies at Temple University, where she is now an Adjunct Professor. She is an annual presenter for a world-renowned mental health conference, as well as a projected presenter for an Ivy League university.

For more information about **Reverse the Adverse** or to have Nicole speak at your organization, please email her at:

nt@theurbanschoolpsychologist.com

Nydia Guity has been in the field of behavioral health since 2011 and has experience working with children, adolescents and older adults in overcoming symptoms of anxiety and depression. Ms. Guity works in an outpatient primary care setting in Atlanta, Georgia servicing clients in addressing mental health needs on the short-term basis with Solution Focused Therapy (SFT).

Ms. Guity also works as an assessment coordinator for children who are survivors of commercial sexual exploitation (CSEC).

Visit www.yournaturalhairapist.com to stay in touch with Ms. Guity.

Catrece Davis is a Licensed Clinical Social Worker, mentor, speaker, and author. She is licensed in the State of Arkansas where she provides mental health services to children, teens, young adults, and their families.

Catrece is a school-based therapist currently working with teens and is passionate about children; desiring to see them flourish beyond their pain and WIN. Her childhood experiences caused her to develop a heightened level of empathy for others, and she has always wanted to help people; leading her into the field of Social Work.

Having earned her Bachelors of Social Work degree in 2005, Catrece then furthered her education and earned a Masters of Social Work degree in 2012.

To contact Catrece, email her at: catrecedavis71@gmail.com

Victoria Miller is a PhD. candidate at Northcentral University and serves as a Non-Commissioned Officer in the United States Army. Her area of study is in Marriage and Family Therapy; specializing in therapy with Military Families. As an aspiring marriage and family therapist, she lets theory and research inform her work and strives to *do no harm* by undergoing extensive training.

Victoria has acquired knowledge and skills centered on cultural dimensions in the family system and how it affects their internal and external functioning. Her passion for the further development of the field has been recognized by Delta Kappa, International Marriage and Family Therapy Honor Society.

In addition to being a scholar-practitioner, Victoria is an Academic Life Coach. She prides herself on being a lifelong learner and provides effective and proven educational coaching to students that changes the way they approach their academic journey.

When she is not knee-deep in her studies, she is a doting wife, mother, and active member of Kappa Epsilon Military Sorority, Inc. Her dedicated service and mentorship to others is the driving force behind her personal and professional life.

You can reach Victoria at:

Email: victoria@infinitealc.com
Website: www.infinitealc.com

As a survivor of child sexual abuse, **Renetta Weaver** lived in a mental fog of depression and was angry. For most of her teen and adult life, she struggled with slow suicide by escaping through emotional eating which ultimately turned into food addiction.

In her despair of carrying the emotional and physical weight that was rooted in guilt and shame, Renetta believed that there was no escape from the cycle of relationship trauma and drama that she experienced. Therefore, earning her Master's Degree in Social Work was a journey of learning and personal healing.

Renetta is now a Licensed Clinical Social Worker, a Master Addictions Counselor and the Clinical Director of a Co-occurring Addictions Program with the Military, and through her work of providing therapy to individuals, families, and groups, Renetta has been able to turn her pain into purpose.

For more information about self-care, overcoming emotional eating, and food addiction, for yourself or your group, please explore her website at www.renettaweaver.com and join her Facebook Community "What's Eating You???"

Ashlee C. Fowlkes is a Licensed Clinical Psychologist. His passion for LGBTQ+ sensitivity is palpable and has resulted in him becoming a highly sought-after speaker and consultant. Having worked in the field of Diversity and Inclusion for the past ten years, Dr. Fowles has been called upon to provide training and consultation to organizations both large and small.

In addition to facilitating training and providing consultation, he will occasionally agree to serve as the keynote speaker at an event. Two examples come to mind. Dr. Fowlkes served as the Keynote speaker at a PRIDE event within the Federal Bureau of Prisons delivering a speech of hope and resilience to openly gay and transgender inmates. And, he was also honored to be selected to deliver the keynote address at Virginia State University's first-ever Lavender Ceremony.

This event proved to be historic as it was the first Lavender Ceremony to be held at an HBCU in the Commonwealth of Virginia.

As a transgender man himself, Dr. Fowlkes has a profound appreciation for the impact (both blatant and subtle) of cultural competence and sensitivity in the workplace. He is considered a subject matter expert and provides consultation on the creation and implementation of policies and procedures related to sexual and/or gender minorities.

Contact Information:

Email: booking@fowlkes.consulting
Website: www.fowlkes.consulting

Daphne Fuller is the founder of Therapeutic Solutions and Wellness, PC and creator of Black Minds in Meditation. She has a private practice and global integrating her work as a Licensed Professional Counselor, Certified Yoga Instructor, Life Coach, Reiki Practitioner and Speaker. She is also collaborating with Fayetteville State University's Collaborative Institute; offering yoga and counseling for veterans and students.

Daphne has a Bachelor of Arts in Psychology with a minor in Child and Family Development from Georgia Southern University and a Master of Arts in Counseling from Webster University - Myrtle Beach campus. She previously worked as a School Counselor and Special Education Teacher for a total of 13 years.

Knowing personally how depression and anxiety can affect your life, Daphne's passion lies in helping adults find their light, and shed old limiting beliefs and circumstances that affect their current state of being. She helps individuals and groups tap into the core of what holds them back while providing emotional support, psycho-education, and tools to maneuver through the process.

Daphne also provides the integration of coaching or counseling with yoga (upon request) to adults. Daphne has spoken about Mental Wellness and Stress Management at churches and provided yoga workshops at hospitals, women's retreats in corporate settings and youth centers.

Web-based services are available. You can contact Daphne at daphnefuller@therapeuticandwellness.com and visit her website at therapeuticandwellness.com

Linda A. Lewter is a Licensed Professional Counselor specializing in Imago Therapy, Solution Focused Therapy, and Cognitive-Behavioural Therapy, among others. Linda's goal in working with individuals is to focus on their relationships with others, uncover unconscious thoughts and drivers, help them regulate their emotions, bring healing in areas of childhood wounding and help them understand how emotions and memories shape them today.

What makes Linda's service distinctive is her uncanny ability to meet client's where they are and help them achieve a positive result in a short number of sessions.

She has worked with individuals, couples, parents and teens, military families, and those caring for aging parents.

Linda received her Bachelor of Science degree from Virginia State University in Petersburg, VA, where she majored in Accounting. She then went on to obtain her Master of Arts degree in Counseling/Psychology from Regent University in Virginia Beach, VA.

Linda lives in the Hampton Roads Virginia area, and when she is not working, she likes to spend time at the beach, reading and spending time with family and friends.

Linda can be contacted at: www.lindalewterlpc.com

Reginald V. Cunningham, Sr. stands at the forefront of the counseling arena. He has spent the past 18 years dedicated to changing the lives of adolescent young men and adults suffering from an array of mental and emotional health and life challenges. He has become a sought-after therapist in the area of Couples and Marriage counseling. Most importantly, he is currently making his mark with bringing attention to the importance of mental health in the Black community through advocacy on local and national stages, helping to reduce the stigma that has kept us void of seeking proper help; particularly among African American men.

Dr. Cunningham is a graduate of Tennessee State University with a Bachelor of Science in Psychology, and received a master's from Coppin State University and Doctorate of Counseling Psychology with an emphasis in Counselor Education and Supervision from Argosy University.

He is a member the American Counselor Association, Black Therapists Rock, and sits on the Prince George's County Mental Health Advisory Committee, where decisions of mental health matters are decided in the southern Maryland area. He is also a member of Kappa Alpha Psi Fraternity, Inc.

More information about Dr. Cunningham can be found on his website at: <u>rvcounseling.com</u> or by email: regisbak@gmail.com

Paula S. Langford is a native Baltimorean. She earned her Master of social work degree from the University of Maryland. In 2000 and 2002 respectively, she became the first African American Roman Catholic female to earn her master and doctorate degrees from Howard University School of Divinity. She is a Corporator at St. Ambrose Catholic Church in Northwest, Baltimore and works in the Northwest Baltimore community to improve community wellbeing.

For the past thirty years, she has worked as a clinical social worker for the District of Columbia and Baltimore City. She is a certified African-centered social work practitioner through the National Association of Black Social Worker's Academy of African Centered Social Work. Dr. Langford is a Sex Health in Recovery facilitator, Certified Problem Gambling facilitator, Reiki Master/Teacher, and Trauma Systems Theory (TST) practitioner. She is currently a Lead Case Practice Specialist/ Child Federal Reviewer for the District of Columbia.

Dr. Langford integrates spirituality and Complementary Alternative Medicine (CAM) social work practices in therapeutic and faith-based settings. She was an adjunct professor at Morgan State University's School of Social Work for nineteen years.

She is passionate about the healing of God's children and families everywhere, and is an advocate for justice, believing that no one is free until we are all free.

Lennie J. Carter, a New York native, credits his upbringing in Brownsville, an underserved community in Brooklyn, as the backdrop for most of his benevolent work; which includes mentorship and spearheading community initiatives.

Black Therapists Rock is one of the many organizations in which Lennie holds a leadership role; assisting over 20,000 mental health practitioners worldwide.

Lennie has procured two degrees from Stony Brook University, a Bachelor of Science in Business Management, and a Master of Science in Human Resources Management. His curriculum vitae reads as someone who has always been strategic in both planning and executing his goals, whether collegiate or entrepreneurial.

Winning an NYC Mayor's award, Lennie has partnered with his investors, Lupe Fiasco and Di-Ann Eisnor, to become an integral figure in the mental health tech industry.

You can find Lennie on social media @lcarterny when he is not learning from his two sons, LJ and Lathan Carter, and teaching them how to be Kings!

Chasity Chandler is a Licensed Mental Health Counselor with several specialization and certifications to increase knowledge and skills to assist her clients. With over 16 years of experience in the helping field, she specializes in working with children, teenagers, and adults on general mental health, trauma, sex/sexuality issues, and substance abuse. Chasity works extensively with the LGBTQ+ population on, and not limited to, the following areas: general therapy around daily concerns, coming out, gender therapy, hRt consideration, and letters, support with family/partners, advocacy and more!

She does a lot of work with couples in areas of communication, conflict resolution, increase intimacy and passion in their relationship as well as infidelity and more! Chasity is currently a Qualified Supervisor for Mental Health Counseling Interns.

In addition to counseling, Chasity is a speaker and offers coaching, consultation, and supervision to other professionals and entrepreneurs. She provides authenticity coaching and is a Certified Daring Way Facilitator; experiential methodology based on the research of Dr. Brené Brown. Chasity also offers training in LGBTQ+ Terminology, LGBTQ+ Cultural Inclusivity and How to Create A Sex-Positive Environment.

You may reach Chasity Chandler by visiting her website at: www.centerforsexualhealthandwellness.com

Founder and President, Deran Young, created Black Therapists Rock (BTR) as she noticed a gap in mental health awareness/community outreach and support for helping professionals. She saw this as an opportunity to organize community leaders, personal development experts, and clinical professionals towards ACTION in decreasing the stigma and other barriers to the mental and emotional well-being within marginalized communities.

Established in 2016, with a vision to elevate the conversation around Black Mental Health to a national platform that creates innovative resources and opportunities for healing, BTR has become a network of over 21,000 professionals!

To find out more about us or to become a member, visit us at:

www.blacktherapistsrock.com

CPSIA information can be obtained
at www.ICGtesting.com
Printed in the USA
BVHW060815010319
541510BV00002B/3